natural living
cosmetics

Lorraine Sutton

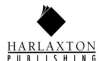

HARLAXTON
PUBLISHING

FRONT JACKET:
Nature provides us with essential herbs, flowers and essences that are akin to the skin, thereby promoting health and healing.

PAGE 2:
Choosing the correct colours to suit your skin undertones will give you confidence, enabling you to feel happy and comfortable about yourself.

Measurements
All spoon measurements are level.
As the imperial/metric/US equivalents are not exact, follow only one system of measurement.

Ingredients
Fresh herbs are used unless otherwise stated. If they are unavailable, use half the quantity of dried herbs.

Published by Harlaxton Publishing Limited
2 Avenue Road, Grantham, NG31 6TA, United Kingdom
A Member of The Weldon International Group of Companies

First published 1994
© 1994 Copyright Harlaxton Publishing Ltd
© 1994 Copyright design Harlaxton Publishing Ltd

Publishing Manager: Robin Burgess
Project Coordinator: Barbara Beckett
Designer: Amanda McPaul
Illustrations: Amanda McPaul
Photographers: Jill White and Ray Jarratt
Typesetting: Sellers, Grantham
Reproduction: G A Graphics, Stamford
Printing: Imago Singapore

British Library Cataloguing-in-Publication data
A catalogue record for this book is available from the British Library
ISBN: 1-85837-060-4

Acknowledgements
Tony Stone Worldwide Photolibrary – pages 2, 10, 27, 44
Picture Bank Photo Library Ltd – pages 13, 46, 47, 49
Britstock-IFA Ltd – page 40

We would like to thank Paul Penders, who freely supplied the natural cosmetics, and the models Clare Hunstead and Amanda McPaul, for taking part in this book

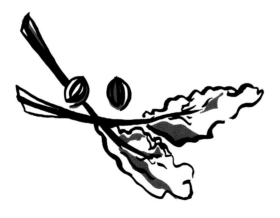

Contents

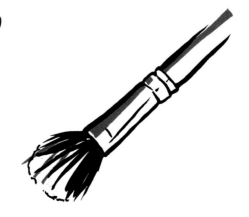

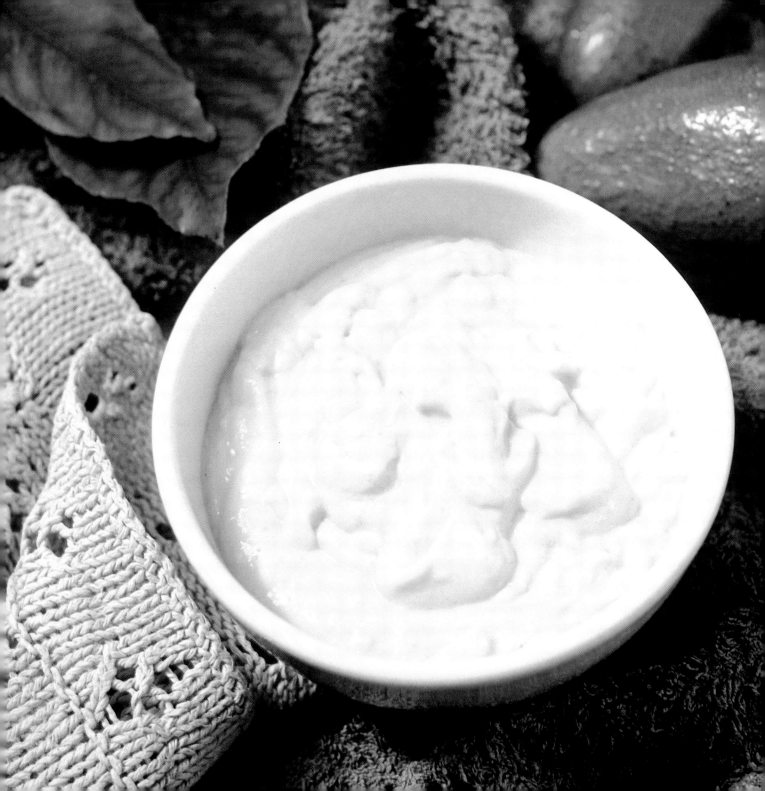

Introduction

*T*he word cosmetics is derived from a Greek word meaning to arrange or put in order. A good cosmetic allows the skin to function in harmony with both the inner you and the outer environment. This truly reinforces the idea that how we look is more than surface appearances. We all want to look good and we use cosmetics to enhance our individual qualities. You will look your best if you take a natural approach, nurturing your skin and giving it a chance to perform its many functions. Deep cleansing, proper protection, gentle exercise, a balanced diet and fresh air will ensure that the skin will regenerate at its fullest capacity.

This book contains a simple introduction to understanding your skin – that fascinating organ that makes such a dynamic contribution to your health as well as your appearance. We explain how to make homemade cosmetics from natural ingredients for your face and hair, using quick and easy recipes you can create in the kitchen. To help you to make the most of your best features, we provide pointers on the choice and application of make-up. We explain the benefits of using the environmentally friendly and cruelty-free products that encourage normal skin functions rather than risking the harmful effects of artificial preservatives, colourings and fragrances.

There is a chapter on protective cosmetics for different environments and another on recognizing and responding to the different skin conditions you can experience from time to time. If you want to look good the natural way, this book will show you how!

OPPOSITE:
Avocado has beneficial soothing and nourishing properties for blemished skin. Try the Avocado mask recipe on page 28.

Understanding Your Skin

Y our skin varies constantly in response to the inner and outer worlds. Different rhythms of the body and the environment will have a direct effect upon it. The skin is the largest organ of the body, and is the only organ exposed to the outside world. The skin on your face is exposed to the elements all year round and adapts itself to different climatic conditions. It also mirrors changes in the body.

OPPOSITE:
Your face is a clear reflection of your whole body as well as your state of mind – past and present.

STRUCTURE OF THE SKIN:
The skin is the largest organ of the body and has many important functions to perform. This diagram shows the most important features of its complex structure.

1   *Horny layer*
2   *Epidermis*
3   *Dermis*
4   *Subcutaneous tissue*
5   *Hair shaft*
6   *Keratin*
7   *Hair follicle*
8   *Sweat duct*
9   *Sebaceous gland*
10   *Papilla*
11   *Inner root sheath*
12   *Arrector pili muscle*
13   *Nerve endings and blood supply*
14   *Collagen fibres*
15   *Basal cells migrate to 1*

H ealthy skin will change regularly, indicating that it is fulfilling its functions of protection, elimination, absorption and heat regulation. The food we put into our bodies has an influence on the skin's health. What we apply to the skin is just as important – latest tests have discovered that chemical substances may be found in the urine within 30 minutes of application to the skin. It is important to nurture the skin and encourage harmony by adopting an holistic approach, that is by treating the skin as an integral part of the whole body.

The role of skin

S kin encloses the whole body in a protective sheath, holding in internal organs and tissue and providing a defence against the outside elements. The skin is made up of three layers, the epidermis, the dermis (true skin) and the subcutaneous layers. (See the illustration below.)

The skin is engaged in a constant process of regeneration over a cycle of about 28 days. Within the living epidermis, new cells from the base (basal cells) are being formed all the time. They take 14 days to migrate to the skin surface, losing water and undergoing chemical changes on the way.

There can be 20 layers or so of dead cells built up in the top (or horny) layer of the epidermis at any one time, providing the body's first defence against infection and foreign bodies. Water cannot penetrate this layer but oil-soluble substances can dissolve in the sebum (oil) that surrounds each hair follicle. These cells remain in the horny layer for 14 days until they are naturally sloughed off as more cells push forward, completing the 28-day cycle. This process is assisted by proper cleansing and hygiene which enable some flaky skin cells to be removed on a daily basis.

The dermis, lying under the epidermis, contains the nerves that feed information to the brain about textures and temperatures, pleasure and pain, allowing you to respond quickly and appropriately to the environment.

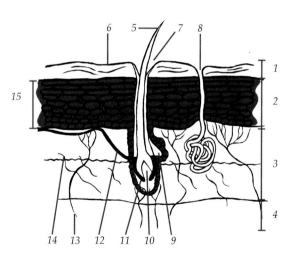

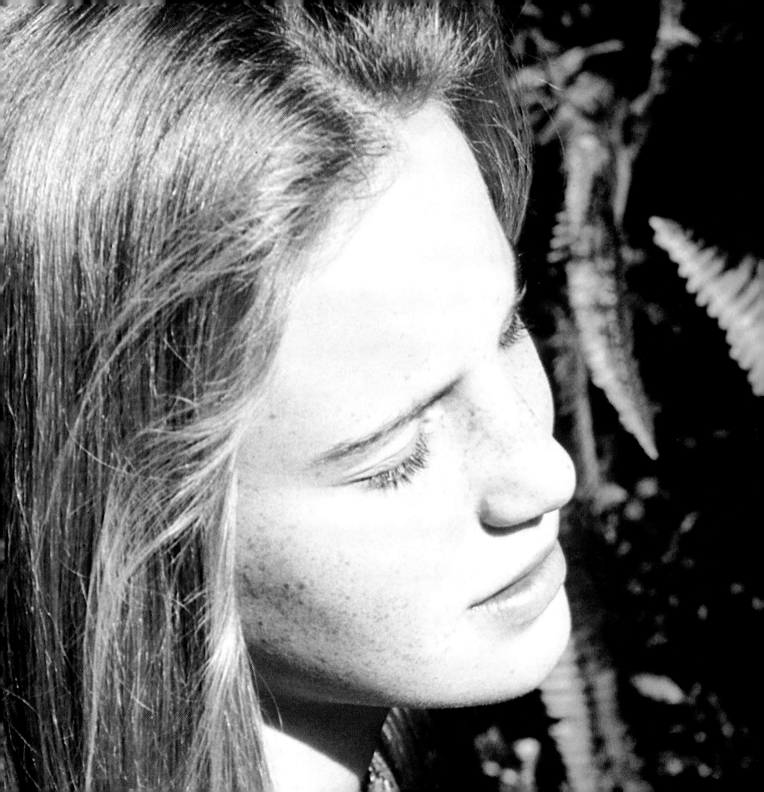

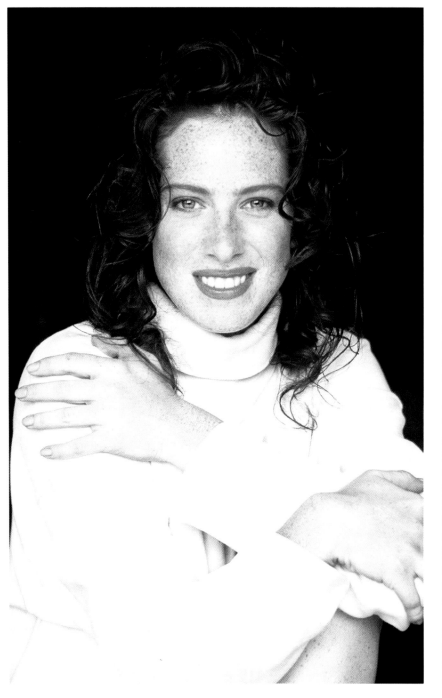

The dermis is fed by the blood capillaries it contains. The skin retains body fluids or releases them through the sweat glands in the dermis in order to maintain a constant body temperature. Perspiration is a combination of water, salts and other chemicals, released by the sweat glands in response to high temperatures. Under normal conditions, the water content of the skin is higher than that of surrounding air, so evaporation occurs from the skin's surface, cooling the body.

A thin layer of sebum (oily, waxy material) is produced by the sebaceous glands in the dermis. Sebum keeps the skin waterproof and resistant to extremes of temperature, minor injuries, chemically active substances and many germs. One or more sebaceous glands is attached to each hair follicle, secreting the sebum to lubricate the skin and preserve the softness of the hair. They are located on all parts of the body except the palms of the hands and the soles of the feet.

The dermis itself is made up of connective tissue which consists of the fibres collagen and elastin. There are more of these fibres in the skin of the face than in the whole of the rest of the body. These fibres link the dermis to the epidermis and to the underlying subcutaneous layers. Collagen is a major protein in elastic fibres, tendons and ligaments and becomes more brittle as you age. Collagen gives tissue elasticity and resistance to pressure, allowing the skin to store water. With age, collagen becomes inelastic, insoluble and rigid, affecting the skin's ability to store water (we are made up of 70 per cent water!) and causing skin to become thinner, drier and more brittle.

The underlying subcutaneous layer (adipose tissue) is located between the dermis and the internal body and comprises closely packed cells containing fat. This layer acts as an insulating buffer (preventing direct heat loss from within the body), provides the shape of body contours and enables the skin to be mobile. The thickness will differ in different parts of the body and from person to person.

The lymph system

The lymph system is a series of articulated vessels which run alongside the blood vessels, but are not connected with them. Lymph fluid is a clear flowing liquid between the skin and muscle. Unlike blood, which is kept moving by the pumping of the heart, lymph relies on the flexibility and condition of the muscles to keep it flowing. The lymph system flows around the body, passing through lymph nodes at many locations. Lymph is essential to supply the skin with food and remove waste products.

The uninterrupted circulation of lymph is important. When a lymph node becomes blocked with an accumulation of toxins, nourishment of the skin is inhibited, and waste materials cannot be released, causing toxicity. Sometimes areas of skin will become problematic around blocked lymph nodes and, since the lymph system is also responsible for distributing weight evenly around the body, blockages can lead to localized weight problems.

The importance of healthy blood for the skin is underestimated. It brings nourishment from the food we eat to the skin via our lymphatic system.

The skin's pH

The body needs to have a balance of acid and alkaline in the blood for good health. A normal skin is about 5.6 on the pH scale, which is slightly more acidic than neutral. A slightly acidic rating guards the skin against bacteria. When skin becomes oily, the pH will be about 4.5 which is on the more acidic side of the scale. The pH of alkaline skin condition is between 6.9 and 9 and can be caused by too much perspiration or by the use of caustic products such as soap, causing a dry skin condition.

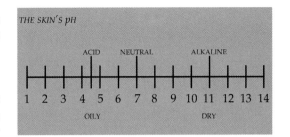

THE SKIN'S pH

	ACID	NEUTRAL	ALKALINE	

1 2 3 4 5 6 7 8 9 10 11 12 13 14

OILY   DRY

OPPOSITE:
Keep skin vital and glowing by using natural treatments and preparations. Make-up will appear more radiant if your skin is clean and healthy.

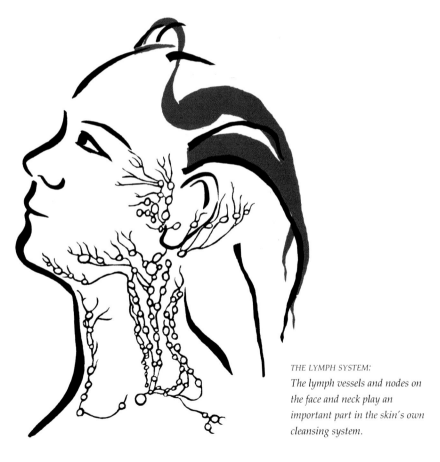

THE LYMPH SYSTEM:
The lymph vessels and nodes on the face and neck play an important part in the skin's own cleansing system.

OPPOSITE:

Healthy skin is a reflection of a healthy mind and body. Enhance healthy skin by choosing make-up colours and tones to suit your particular skin undertone (see Skin undertones, page 42).

CHINESE FACIAL CHART:

The Chinese facial chart shows how problem areas on the face can give an indication of imbalances in different parts of the body.

1   *Bladder*
2   *Small intestine*
3   *Spleen*
4   *Liver*
5   *Bladder*
6   *Sleep centre*
7   *Kidneys*
8   *Respiratory organs – lungs*
9   *Heart*
10   *Intestines*
11   *Pancreas*
12   *Hormonal – sexual*
13   *Gall bladder*
14   *Uterus*
15   *Liver region*
16   *Stomach*
17   *Adrenals*
18   *Pancreas*
19   *Large intestine*

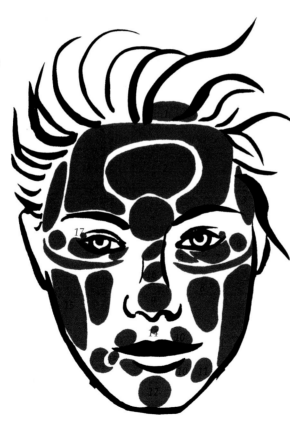

Skin as an indicator

Changes to the skin are occurring all the time throughout life and are influenced by weather and the seasons, growth phases, the general condition of the body and mind and the amount of tender loving care you give yourself. Skin will react differently from one person to another. Healthy skin can be achieved by self-awareness and knowing how to respond correctly to signs of imbalance (see page 54). You can improve your self-awareness by simply examining your skin closely in the mirror each morning, and reading the story your face tells.

Your face is a reflection of your whole body. Look out for changes such as dark circles under the eyes, weight problems, puffiness, recurring blemishes, pimples, blackheads, flakiness, dryness, oiliness or wrinkles. These can be indications of imbalance within the body or a sign of mishandling. You need to encourage the skin to normalize. Sometimes this can be done by changing your diet slightly or including more exercise and relaxation in your lifestyle. (See the Chinese facial chart opposite to discover what areas of the body may need attention.)

Skin colouring can vary, especially when you have eaten too much of a particular food. The colours themselves can be helpful indications: for example, white can mean over-consumption of dairy products; red may indicate the heart is working overtime; brown may signal gall bladder and liver problems.

It is common for people to be self-conscious about the appearance of their skin, especially on the face, for the face is the most expressive part of the body. It is also the focus of other people's attention. After all, it is the chief way human beings recognize each other – there is even a part of the human brain specifically dedicated to the recognition of faces. Your face is the clearest reflection of your state of mind, past and present. Grief, anger, fear, depression, joy, laughter can all literally leave their mark on your skin, especially from around your mid-30s – so take care you are not habitually frowning or screwing up your face!

The skin as a sense organ

Skin is the largest sense organ and is thinner on the face, where it protects other sense organs such as the eyes, ears, nose and mouth. Our senses carry messages through the central nervous system to the brain, reporting on the world around us, so that we may guide, nourish and protect ourselves.

The senses remain healthy by being active. When was the last time you enjoyed sitting in a fragrant garden, felt the grass under your feet, or listened to the wind blowing through the trees? The elements of nature provide endless stimulation to the senses, satisfying our hunger for beauty and pleasure.

Avoid abusive cleansing ingredients and certain peeling and scrubbing techniques. They will damage the protective acid mantle of the skin. Electrical impulses used on the skin, hot and cold temperature fluctuations, sun abuse, and chemically prepared skincare products can weaken the skin's metabolism, breaking down its natural responsiveness. Many people have become totally dependent on artificial cosmetics, using substitution therapy rather than support therapy. If you use natural ingredients that are akin to the skin, they will gently exercise the use of your senses. The energy exchange will strengthen the responsiveness of your skin and promote the regeneration process of the body. Learn to distinguish between a substitution therapy and a support therapy.

Now that you understand more about the skin, you will be in a better position to nurture it sensitively, to support its essential work. In return, your skin will reward you, giving you the glow of someone in harmony with the inner and outer worlds.

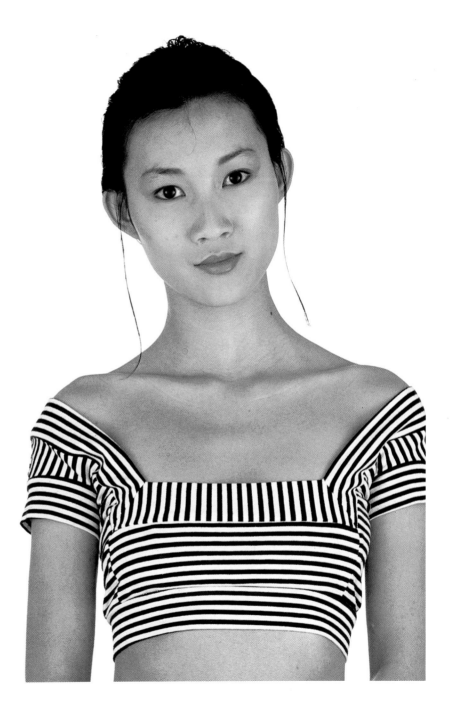

Homemade Preparations

When applying cosmetics, make sure they are as gentle and pure as possible. Finding genuinely natural and safe products is not an easy task, however, especially when there is no legal definition of the word 'natural'. Truly natural cosmetics contain renewable ingredients, preferably grown using biodynamic or organic gardening methods, or grown in their natural surroundings. Look for ingredients that are free of petrochemicals and synthetic fragrances and that do not pollute the environment during their manufacture and use.

Fresh, living ingredients give the skin a wonderful alive feeling. Working with the textures, colours and aromas of plants is a healing experience in itself and will exercise your senses. Be aware that there are many misleading claims surrounding natural cosmetics. Many products will include only small amounts of natural-sounding products that lose their active properties during heavy processing methods. Some ingredients are stressful to the skin and can place too many demands upon the skin's cell structure – these include colours, fragrances, mineral oils, talc, glycols, phenol, formaldehyde, to name a few. Always check labels and do not be afraid to ask about ingredients you are not sure of.

Animal testing is being discouraged within the cosmetics industry and a number of successful alternative testing methods now exist. Many people are becoming committed to this cause as they learn about the cruel experiments that animals have been, and still are, subjected to for the testing of cosmetics. Products marked 'cruelty-free' usually have not been tested on animals.

Making cosmetics

Cooking experience can be a help in deciding what combinations are good and what consistencies work well, but follow your instincts when preparing your cosmetics.

Choose fresh, seasonal and high-quality ingredients and raw materials, to ensure greater effect and a longer shelf life. Use the ingredients that appeal to you most – more than likely they are what your skin condition requires. If you start off your homemade cosmetics by trying simple recipes with ingredients that you know well, you'll have more confidence using them. You will gradually experiment more with other ingredients.

Learn to understand the properties of your ingredients – for example, whether they are a good emulsifier or stabilizer or whether they will have a warming or cooling effect. You may be surprised to find that some of the simplest mixtures often give the best results. So, relax and follow your intuition. If you are really unsure about an ingredient, do a patch test to look for any possible reaction or leave that ingredient out altogether. Your cupboards will eventually build up quite a selection of ingredients from which to choose, enabling you to become more creative as time goes on.

OPPOSITE:

It is important to choose fresh, high-quality ingredients when preparing your homemade cosmetics so that your skin can benefit fully from their active properties.

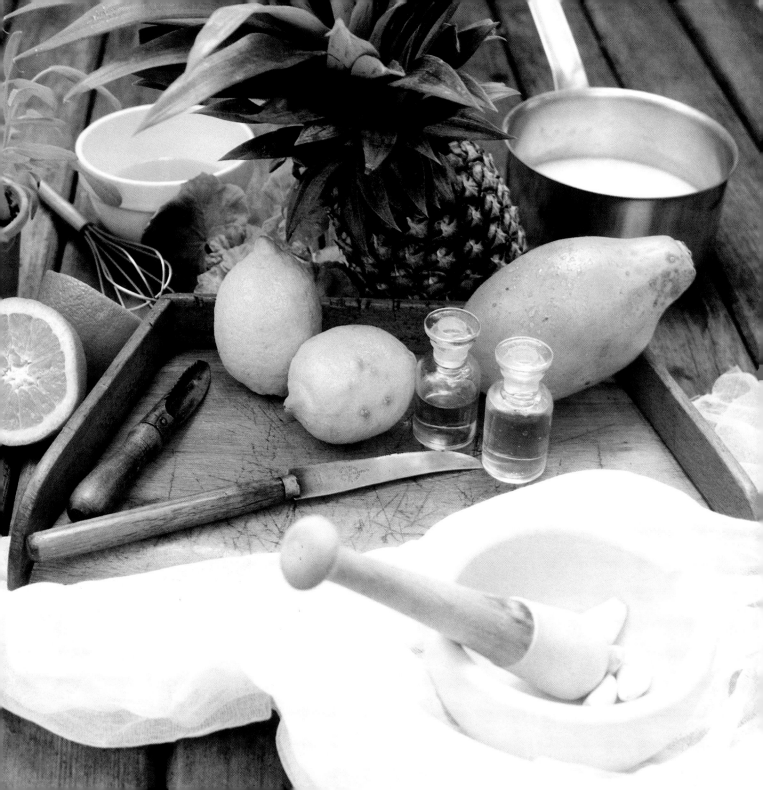

What you will need

Basic kitchen equipment such as a double saucepan (boiler – although an enamel bowl in a saucepan will suffice), pestle and mortar, mixer, egg whisk, wire sieves (strainers), funnels, a selection of enamel, china or stainless steel bowls, jugs (pitchers), measuring spoons, scales, muslin/cheesecloth for filtering (this may be substituted by an unbleached coffee filter bag) and sterilized jars for storing your homemade cosmetic preparations.

Although electrical equipment is often more convenient, it is preferable that hand-refining methods are used in order to preserve and enhance the properties of the natural ingredients.

This chapter introduces some very easy and effective preparation recipes that are the foundation of many products sold on the market. Here we will use natural ingredients instead of the synthetic alternatives. If you can get back to the basics and use pure, natural ingredients, your skin and body will benefit and be much healthier.

Some basic cosmetic chemistry

Oil (sebum) and water are naturally present in the skin, helping the skin to remain soft and supple. As our body ages, production of oil decreases and the skin becomes drier. Creams are blends of oil and water called emulsions. Creams are separated into two categories, depending on their oil-to-water ratio. See the illustration below.

An oil-in-water emulsion is one where very small oil droplets are surrounded by a continuous body of water – milk, for example. The smaller the droplets are, the more stable the emulsion. Emulsifying agents are often added to improve stability. In general, an oil-in-water emulsion has a more creamy texture and a water-in-oil emulsion feels greasy.

The effects of the two emulsions are quite different. The evaporation of the water from an oil-in-water emulsion applied to the skin causes a refreshing sensation and leaves a thin film of oil, which prevents moisture loss. A water-in-oil emulsion lets the oil contact the skin surface immediately. Because the water evaporation is inhibited by the oil, it is not as refreshing.

A SOLUTION – is made by dissolving one substance (solute) into another (solvent). They do not require an emulsifier as they dissolve with each other, for example an essential oil mixed into a carrier oil.

A SUSPENSION – is a mixture of insoluble powders in a liquid medium and needs to be shaken before use. It is made by mixing small amounts of water into the powder to form a smooth paste, then the balance of the liquid is added. For example, cleansing grains mixed with water.

EMULSIONS:

An oil-in-water emulsion (left) and a water-in-oil emulsion (right).

1   Oil
2   Water

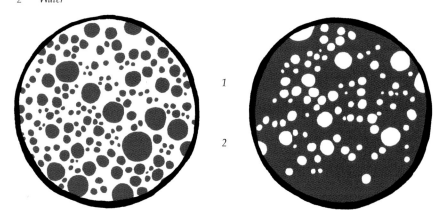

Cleanser, toner and moisturizer

To ensure that your skin is looking its best at all times, you need to deep cleanse, tone and protect it. Homemade preparations will promote the healthy function of the skin.

Cleanser

There are many ways to cleanse your skin. It is preferable to deep cleanse using a water-in-oil emulsion which is able to penetrate deep into the pores to dissolve grease and remove accumulated grime from below the surface. Water completes the cleansing process by removing dust and water-soluble salts left on the skin by perspiration.

An oil-in-water emulsion will only remove surface make-up and grime. It can be used on a sensitive skin suffering from excessive dryness or allergic reactions. When the skin is dry, sensitive or blemished, oil cannot penetrate very well, so soften the skin first by soaking with warm water, loosening the dead surface cells.

To apply cleansing cream, dab it on to five to seven points of the face, then spread over the skin with fingertips, avoiding the eye area. Compress your skin, using moist, cupped hands in a suction movement, making sure grains never scrape the skin. Splash the face with warm water to remove all traces.

Cleansing milks can be applied in the same manner or by using cotton wool and lightly spreading over the skin. Rinse off with water. Water is the revitalizing secret of eternal youth.

Soap is not classed as a cosmetic but it can be very convenient. If you find you must use it from time to time, use an unscented, pure vegetable-oil soap, the oilier the better. Avoid 'deodorant' soaps as they can be drying and irritating. Many of these

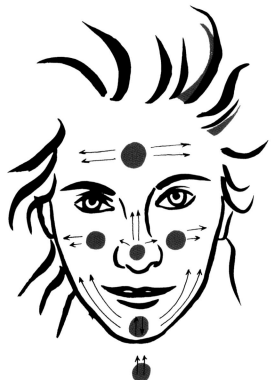

HOW TO APPLY LOTION:
There are two steps in applying lotions to the face. Step one – dab lotion on to points shown. Step two – spread lotion evenly and very lightly over the face with the fingertips to create as little drag as possible.

tip

An holistic approach to health will have positive effects on your skin – having plenty of sleep, drinking plenty of water, eating nutritious food, and learning to relax will help your skin to do its job.

contain fixatives which allow the scents to stay on the skin all day.

Lather soap with water and apply to the skin, leave it for half a minute and wash off with tepid water, perhaps using compress movements with your hands and fingers to ensure soap is fully removed from pores. Never rub the skin or use hard circular movements over it. Oils are necessary to protect the delicate acid mantle of the skin. Once the acid mantle is damaged, the skin is temporarily unprotected, causing moisture loss, sensitivity and redness. Soap can be a direct cause of this condition.

Toner

Toners are usually almost completely made with water (oil-in-water emulsions). They remove the last traces of make-up and debris by dissolving what is left on the skin. Their use is important for regulating the skin's pH. They are ideal to use during the day to remove an oily film or perhaps just to freshen up the skin. They will not close pores, but they do have a positive influence on restoring the acid mantle, which will have the effect of naturally reducing the size of the pores.

If your skin is sensitive, you may find even the mildest toner too strong. Dampen your cotton wool pad (swab) first with water and squeeze the excess water out, before adding the toner to the pad. You will only need to apply with one sweeping movement over the skin surface. Avoid heavy movements and do not rub the toner in or it may dry the skin.

Moisturizer

Water cannot be put back into the skin. We can only help the skin retain moisture by protecting it with a fine film moisturizer. Moisture will be retained when a protective shield covers the skin.

When caring for your skin during the summer months, and when your skin is perspiring during exercise, your protective shield may only have to be a fine film of light skin oil, such as apricot kernel or jojoba. This coverage will encourage elasticity and prevent toxins and oils clogging your pores. Make sure you drink plenty of water to replenish water lost from the body at these times.

Use a moisturizing milk, or a light cream for oily skin conditions. Younger skins will benefit using this also. Save the heavier moisturizing creams for extra protection from the cold or windy weather conditions, when the air is drier. As skin ages, a richer nourishing cream can help the skin to store water and to hold skin connective tissue in place. When the skin is dehydrated, a richer cream will prevent skin dryness and premature wrinkling, giving the skin more time to reach and maintain its ideal moisture level from within. Take care – a heavier moisturizer on a young or oily skin can result in skin problems.

NIGHT REPAIR – You can inhibit the body's natural ability to regenerate by the use of creams during the night. At night skin needs to rest and release the toxins that have built up in the body. Your skin will produce its own oils and moisture during the night, so you do not really need a cream to do it for you. Your skin should be cleansed and toned without any feeling of dryness on going to bed. If your skin feels dry, apply what is required but lightly compress any excess creams away before sleep. Drink plenty of water – water is the element of life.

Recipes

Cleansers penetrate deep into the pores to dissolve grease and grime from below the surface.

Make-up remover

Almond oil is a very good make-up remover, as is jojoba oil. Dampen a cotton wool pad (swab) with oil and use to remove make-up before cleansing. Avoid getting into eyes.

Cleansing grains

Cleansing grains make a wonderful, gentle cleanser, when combined with lukewarm spring water. Remove all traces of make-up and compress the paste on to the face with moist, cupped hands in a suction movement.

If the skin is sensitive, apply a thin layer of vegetable oil (for example, grapeseed or apricot kernel) to the skin 20 minutes before applying the cleansing grain paste. This softens and loosens dry surface cells.

To prepare cleansing grains, sift meal or flour of your choice and mix with lukewarm spring water to give a thick paste. Try oatmeal, corn meal, barley meal, soya flour, potato flour, ground rice meal, ground almonds and adzuki bean meal.

Vegetable oils may also be added to some cleansing grains to give a softer effect. A pestle and mortar could be useful to grind the meals to a finer, smoother consistency.

Aloe vera and rose-water cold cream

Cold creams are used for cleansing and moisturizing and are suitable for aged skin or dry, allergy-prone skin.

3/4 teaspoon vitamin E oil
2 teaspoons aloe vera gel
3 tablespoons almond oil
1 tablespoon hydrous lanolin
2½ tablespoons rose-water (page 22)

Combine vitamin E oil, almond oil, hydrous lanolin and aloe vera gel in a double saucepan (boiler). Heat and stir until the oils are blended with the gel. Remove from the heat. Add the rose-water slowly, whisking vigorously until it is cool. Apply to the skin, avoiding the eye area.

Yoghurt cleansing milk

This recipe is for an all in one cleanser and toner preparation.

2 tablespoons plain yoghurt
1/2 teaspoon wheatgerm (or grapeseed) oil
2 teaspoons clear honey
2 tablespoons peeled and finely shredded apple
1 teaspoon lemon juice
2 teaspoons potato flour

Mix together the yoghurt, wheatgerm oil, honey, apple and lemon juice. Blend in the potato flour to make a smooth creamy consistency. Apply the mixture with the fingers, using the same method as in the Cleansing grains procedure, or alternatively, apply using a cotton wool pad (swab) and remove excess residue with water.

Herbal moisturizing wash

These are effective cleansing milks. Milk will act as the emollient and the herbs will act according to their properties, for example peppermint will have a cooling and antiseptic effect, camomile will calm and soothe, elder flowers will cleanse an inflamed skin safely.

450 ml/3/4 pint/2 cups of warm milk
2 tablespoons herbs of your choice

Add the milk to herbs in a bowl and steep for 3 hours. Strain the milk and apply to the skin with a cotton wool pad (swab). Rinse the skin, compressing to ensure the complete removal of the milk.

Fruity cleansers

GRAPES – are regarded as a living vital substance, a type of blood in vegetable form. Split large grapes, remove pips and rub the flesh over neck and face. Remove with tepid water.

PINEAPPLE – contains enzymes to rejuvenate and will benefit sluggish, oily skin conditions. Wipe a slice of pineapple over the face and rinse.

Soothing cleanser

2 teaspoons soya oil
1 tablespoon wholemeal soya flour, sifted
1 egg
2 teaspoons camomile tea

Mix all ingredients together well. Use same method of cleansing as with the Cleansing grains (page 19), or leave 3 minutes on skin before rinsing with tepid water.

Almond cleansing paste

This is a gentle deep cleanser that is suitable for all skin types.

2 1/2 tablespoons ground almonds, sifted
1 tablespoon almond oil
1 tablespoon lemon juice
1 drop of rose essential oil, optional
Spring water

Mix almond, oils and lemon juice together and add spring water to give a paste consistency. Apply to face as described above.

Toners remove the last traces of make-up and debris by dissolving what is left on the skin.

Cucumber toner

This is a well-known remedy for cooling and toning a dull and lifeless complexion or an oily skin condition.

1 cucumber, peeled and sliced
3 tablespoons spring water or flower water (page 22)

Mash the cucumber with pestle and mortar, add water or flower water. Strain carefully through clean muslin (cheesecloth). Bottle and refrigerate.

Mineral water

Simply decant the mineral water into a glass spray container and use to freshen the skin during a hot day.

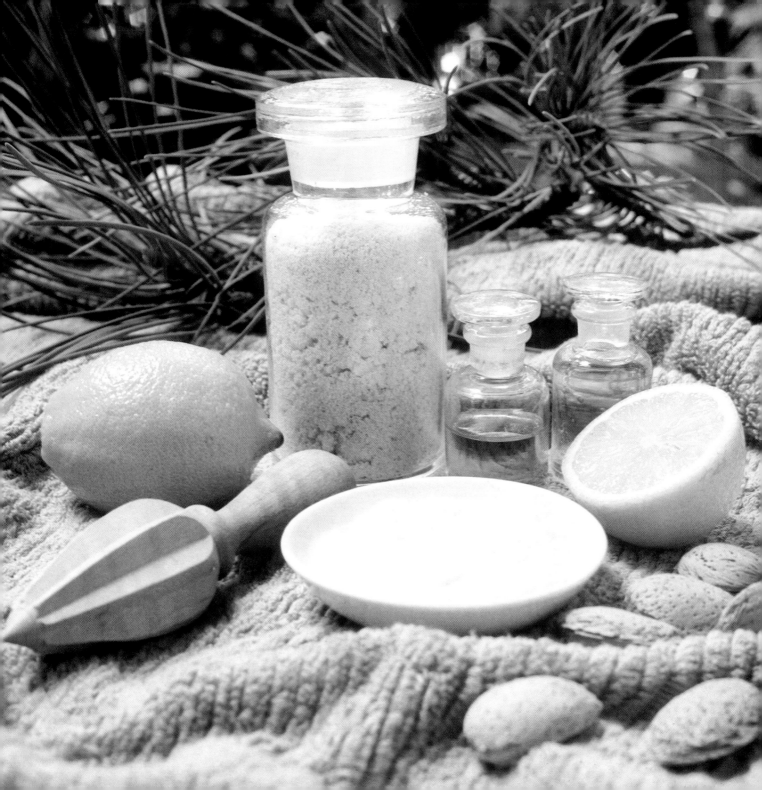

OPPOSITE:
Lime fresh can be easily made from lime and lemon. See the recipe on this page. Splash it on after cleansing.

Flower waters

Flower waters have been used for centuries to harmonize and scent the skin. They are refreshingly simple to make using a selection of fresh rose petals, orange blossom flowers, lavender flowers or violets.

1 large cup fresh (½ cup dried) petals
250 ml/8 fl oz/1 cup boiling water
8 teaspoons vodka, optional

Pour boiling water over the petals, seal and leave for 12–24 hours at room temperature. Then refrigerate for 2 days. Remove from refrigerator and strain. Add vodka and mix. Apply to face with a cotton wool pad (swab) moistened with water. Store in refrigerator.

Herbal toner

Different herbs can be used with water to balance the skin condition and to cleanse. You can brew a single herb or select a small mixture of herbs. Choose a mixture from some examples below.

ACNE – thyme, mint, fennel leaves and seeds, camomile or lavender.
TIRED SKIN – rosemary, nettle, comfrey, camomile.
ALL TYPES – thyme used on its own is an effective toner for all skin conditions.

Cover the selection of your choice (about 2–4 tablespoons) with boiling water, cover and leave to infuse at room temperature for 24 hours. Strain the toner into a bottle and keep refrigerated.

Lime fresh

The combination in this recipe will leave the skin with a cool, tingling feeling.

1 tablespoon lime juice
1 tablespoon lemon juice
1 tablespoon spring water

Mix ingredients and bottle. Refrigerate for storage.

Moisturizers should be applied to a cleansed skin, for about 10 minutes absorption time. Remove any excess with a tissue pressed over the face or a fine film of toner on a cotton wool pad (swab). Wipe the face once only. Moisturizers can be used to soak the skin before a cleanse for better absorption.

Aloe moisture gel

A light moisturizer suitable for young and oilier skin conditions.

5 g/⅙ oz agar agar
250 ml/8 fl oz/1 cup water or St John's Wort tea, strained
2 tablespoons aloe vera gel
1 teaspoon lemon juice
1 tablespoon avocado oil

Soak agar agar for 1 hour in spring water. Strain and squeeze out extra water. Place agar agar in saucepan with water or St John's Wort tea and simmer for 5–10 minutes. Remove from heat and add remaining ingredients. Stir until cold. Store in small, sterile jars in refrigerator. Remove from refrigerator 30 minutes before use. Keeps 2–3 days.

tip

Store your preparations in dark coloured jars, amber or blue for example, to avoid exposure to sunlight and heat, which shorten shelf life. Sterilize your jars for homemade preparations, and when storing in refrigerator, use a few small jars rather than one big one to avoid contamination. Wipe sides clean of ingredients such as oils as they quickly become rancid. Even clean hands carry bacteria.

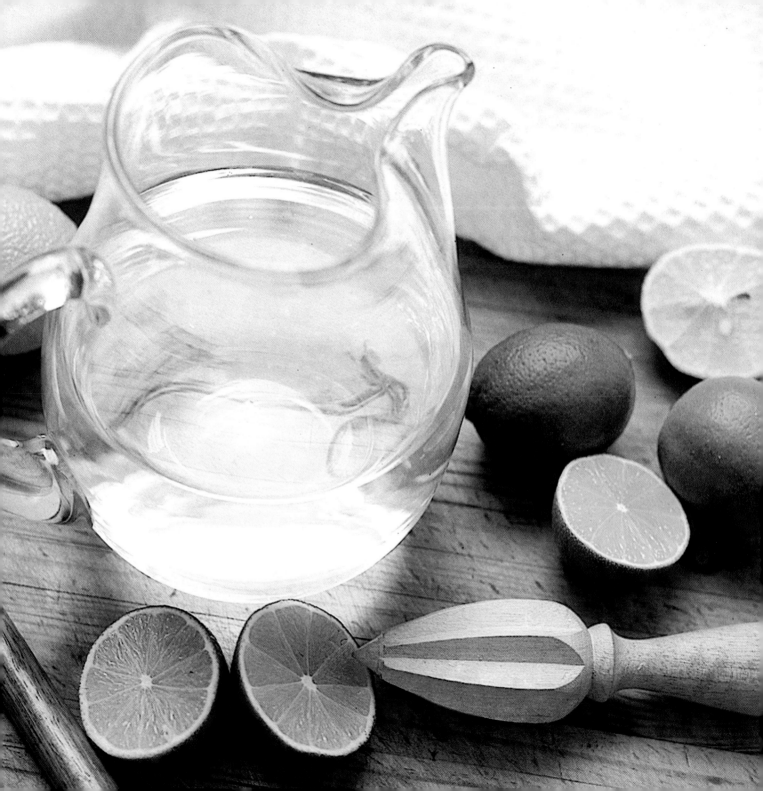

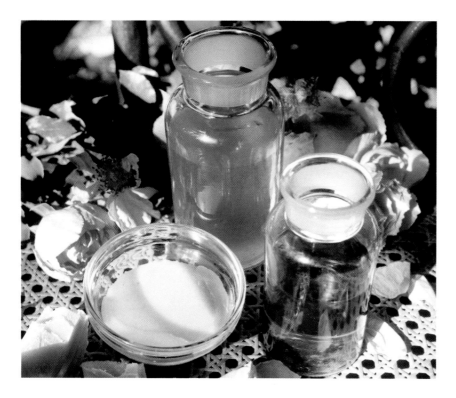

Strawberry face cream

This recipe is particularly suitable for oily skin conditions.

1 tablespoon cocoa butter
4 tablespoons soya oil
1 tablespoon strawberry juice

Melt the cocoa butter in double saucepan (boiler), add soya oil, and mix together. Remove from heat and add strawberry juice, beating until cool. Store in small, sterile glass jars in refrigerator.

Vitamin E cream

This recipe is suitable for dry, damaged skin (chapping, flaking). The Flower water recommended is Orange blossom flower water.

8 tablespoons olive oil
2 tablespoons grated beeswax
4 tablespoons flower water (page 22) or spring water
3/4 teaspoon vitamin E oil

Melt the olive oil and beeswax in a double saucepan (boiler). Remove from heat and stir in orange water. Add the vitamin E oil and stir until cool. Store in small, sterile glass jars in refrigerator.

Rose cream

A soothing, protective cream, suitable for dry, sensitive, mature skins.

1 tablespoon grated beeswax
4 tablespoons olive oil
1–2 tablespoon almond oil
1–2 tablespoon rose-water (page 22)
1–2 drops rose essential oil

Place beeswax, olive oil, almond oil and rose flower water in double saucepan (boiler). Heat and mix well until beeswax has melted. Remove from heat, add essential oil and mix until cool. Store in sterile glass jars in refrigerator.

Oils for skin care

Vegetable oils	Qualities
ALMOND	moisturizing and protective.
APRICOT KERNEL	for elasticity of the skin, especially drying, ageing skin.
AVOCADO	rich in vitamins and sterols, revitalizing.
CARROT	carotene natural source of vitamin A, keeps skin supple, can tend to give skin an orange appearance.
GRAPESEED	light, refreshing, mild astringent qualities.
JOJOBA	obtained from the jojoba bean, similar to human sebum.
SUNFLOWER	extracted from the sunflower seeds, contains essential fatty acids.
VIRGIN OLIVE	obtained from ripe fruit of the olive tree, warming.

Avocado oil is one of the oils that penetrate human skin the most. Jojoba oil has a similar make-up to the structure of sebum, giving extra protection to the skin. Oils can protect the skin from drying, cold weather. Dry, sensitive conditions, however, will need a water-in-oil combination.

Some oils become cloudy in storage, particularly in cold weather. They can be used by themselves or as important ingredients in cosmetic cream mixtures. They have emollient (softening and soothing) properties. Some vegetable oils are lighter than others, for example, jojoba oil is lighter than olive oil.

The following skin conditions can benefit from the suggested essential oils. Vary them as skin condition changes. Always use a carrier cream or oil (such as jojoba or avocado).

Skin	Essential oils
NORMAL	jasmine, lavender, geranium.
DRY	rose, sandalwood, geranium, patchouli, lemon.
MATURE	frankincense, rose, patchouli.
OILY	cypress, juniper, bergamot, lavender, basil, frankincense, cedarwood, lemon.
ACNE	fennel, marjoram, sweet orange juniper.
INFLAMED	camomile, neroli, rose, tangerine, ylang ylang, lavender.

Pure essential oils are natural and come from different parts of plants. These oils are highly concentrated extracts and should not be applied directly to the skin. Always use a carrier oil, or cream base. Provided you avoid essential oils such as bergamot and citrus fragrances which can produce adverse reactions in sunlight, essential oils can bring a sense of joy to your daily skincare regime. You can always investigate the properties of an essential oil in an aromatherapy directory before applying to your skin.

Use only pure, high-quality oils as they achieve therapeutic results. Do not exceed recommended dosages. Add only one or two drops each of your chosen oils to a carrier oil (see above) or a cream base. They make lovely moisturizer creams. Essential oils can also be added to bath water and will make a wonderful compress or inhalation. Essential oils are used in the healing art of aromatherapy.

Seek professional aromatherapists for alternative medicinal treatment. They work holistically and have long-term results on the physical, emotional and spiritual levels.

tip

When removing your cold homemade toners from refrigerator, pre-soak cotton rounds in warm water to take the cold sensation away from skin. For creams, remove from refrigerator 20–30 minutes before use.

Facial Treats

*N*ature has provided a range of clays (red, green, yellow, white and pink) and moor, an organic substance formed naturally from over 400 species of herbs and flowers which have a deep cleansing, toning and restorative action on facial skin and muscles.

Applied to the face, they draw tension and toxins away and remove excess acid from the skin – ideal to maintain and enhance your youthful health and beauty without need of a facial massage.

Facial massage

Facial massage is best avoided. Face muscles are finely tuned for making the most complex movements, such as registering emotion in facial expressions or rapidly forming words. They are not as large or as strong as those in the body, so they can only be stretched slightly. Unlike many muscles of the body that are fixed to bones at both ends, facial muscles are only fixed to bone at one end, the other end being attached to delicate elastic fibres within the dermis layer. Facial massage can easily over-stretch the connective tissue and actually cause sagging and lack of muscle tone.

Only ever use *light* pressure on your face with fingers, even when cleansing or applying creams, and avoid any pulling or pushing of muscles. You will increase and maintain muscle tone by carefully using a firm, light touch across the muscles of the face, rather than downwards.

General exercise, sleep and relaxation for stress management can be useful when you need to release tension build-up in facial muscles. A gentle head or foot massage can have positive results too.

Masks

Masks can be used by all skin conditions to stimulate blood and circulation to promote elimination of waste materials. At the same time, they can also be soothing and moisturizing. Some masks will specifically reduce puffiness and redness and calm blemished skin, others will stimulate. Avoid peel-off masks. For greater effect, steam the skin first, using a mixture of herbs and flowers (see Facial steaming, page 29). Apply masks, after steaming, while the skin is still moist and soft. Leave your mask on for about the same time as you have steamed.

Remember always to protect and soften the eye area, cover broken capillaries and sensitive areas before applying your mask. When a mask starts to harden, remove it. The active ingredients have finished their work and removal soon becomes difficult without hard rubbing. To remove a mask, hold a warm towel against skin to loosen, and gently wipe over the surface, taking care not to use dragging movements. Rinse afterwards with water and always follow with a toner to regulate pH. A normal skin may only need a mask once a month whereas a problem skin will need a mask more regularly to help restore its rhythm.

OPPOSITE:

All skin conditions benefit from regular facial masks. Some masks stimulate the skin, while others soothe and moisturize. See the Yoghurt mask recipe, on page 28, to determine which mask would be beneficial for you.

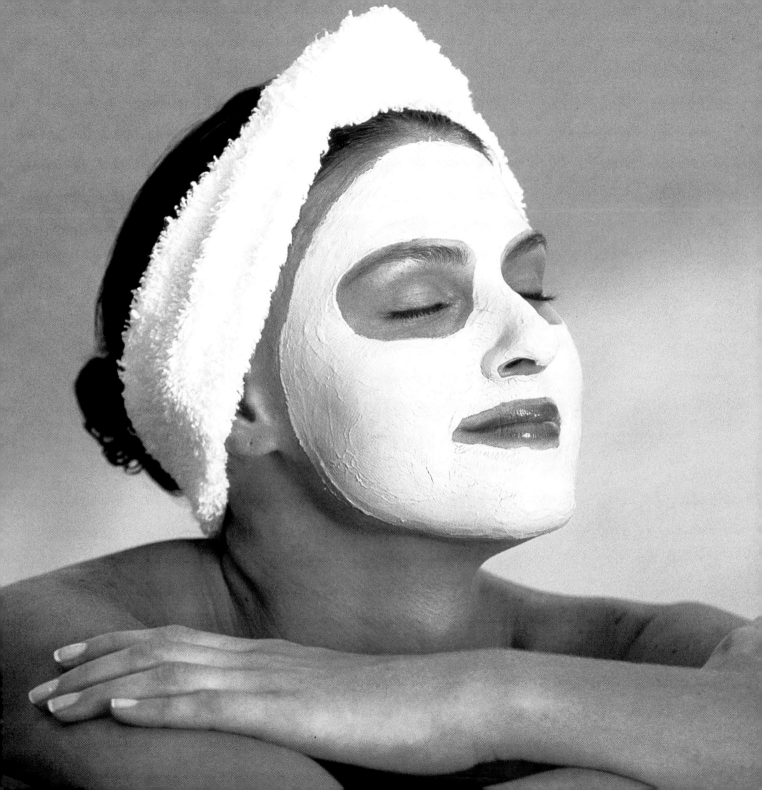

FACE MUSCLES:
The muscles of the face are very delicate and should be treated with care. Unnecessary facial massage or vigorous application of cosmetics can lead to over-stretching and sagging. A light touch is best.

Recipes

Avocado mask

For blemished skin. Purée one ripe avocado and apply as is or combine with an equal amount of soured cream or yoghurt. You can also add 1 tablespoon each of clear honey and olive oil, if you wish.

Buttermilk mask

Suitable for blemished and dry, allergy-prone skins. It restores the acid mantle. Smooth buttermilk over face and neck, and allow to dry. Loosen with a warm to cool compress, rinse with tepid water and blot dry.

Yoghurt mask

Yoghurt has cleansing, toning and extractive properties. Use only plain yoghurt as it contains more active ingredients. Use alone or add it to other ingredients for different effects. Some mixtures will stimulate and others soothe. Use no more than two fruits and no more than two essential oils.

The following skin conditions will benefit from using the suggested ingredients.

Skin	Ingredients
ACNE	brewer's yeast, grape or cabbage juice, tomato, juniper, bergamot.
DRY/MATURE	apples, papaya (pawpaw), avocados, grape juice, bananas, carrots, melons, rose, sandalwood, lemon cypress, patchouli, wheatgerm oil.
HYDRATED	clay, oatmeal or linseed meal, juniper, lavender.
OILY	grape or cabbage juice, tomato, juniper, strawberry, bergamot, lemon juice, pear, frankincense, mashed pineapple.
SENSITIVE	honey, grape, lemon, neroli, rose, camomile.

You will need about 2 parts yoghurt to 1 part fruit or vegetable. Mix your ingredients well and pat on to a clean, moist face. Leave to penetrate for 10–20 minutes, wipe over gently and rinse off with warm water.

Strawberries and cream

2 large strawberries
1 tablespoon cream

Mash together and pat over face and neck. Leave 10–20 minutes. Rinse with tepid water.

tip

Add a dash of milk to your essential oil-in-water. The milk will act as an emulsifier, enabling the oil to mix more readily with the water.

There are hundreds of essential oils available. Always take care with them and be sure to understand their properties before use.

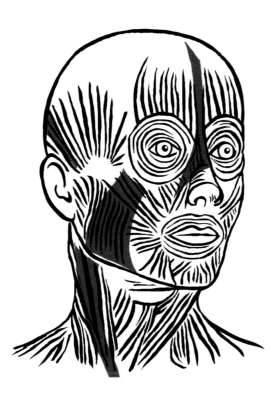

Calendula face mask

1 tablespoon calendula flowers
1 tablespoon camomile flowers
125 ml/4 fl oz/½ cup boiling water
1 tablespoon steamed and mashed carrot
1 teaspoon wheatgerm oil
1 teaspoon almond oil
1 tablespoon soy lecithin granules

Place flowers and boiling water in bowl, stand aside 10–20 minutes. Mix mashed carrot, almond and wheatgerm oil thoroughly. Add flowers and purée. Blend in the lecithin granules to make creamy. Lie back for this one and perhaps lay muslin (cheesecloth) over the face to adhere ingredients.

Pure honey

Dab clear honey on to a blemish or inflamed pimple to draw it out.

Parsley mask

Parsley is rich in iron and is used to normalize a combination skin.

½ cup fresh parsley
1 tablespoon honey
Boiling water

Crush parsley with a mortar and pestle until juice runs out. Mix in honey. Add boiling water to cover. Leave to brew for 20 minutes (until lukewarm) and pat on to face. Place muslin (cheesecloth) over the face to help the mask adhere. This can be warm also if you wish. Leave for 10–15 minutes. Rinse off with tepid water.

Facial steaming

A lovely herbal steam bath, containing blends of herbs, flowers and essential oils, will relax and soften skin. These ingredients mixed with the heat of the steam have an intensive moistening effect as well as being antibacterial. They stimulate the nerve processes and skin secretion. The whole body can benefit from a facial steam as sitting upright and inhaling the vapours will open the lungs. If you find relaxed breathing difficult, apply a warm compress (soaked in the same steam solution) to your back or your neck and shoulders. Breathe slowly in through the nose and out through the mouth at your own pace. Come up for a breather every now and again if you need to. Steaming and deep breathing are a great way to let go. Protect sensitive areas first, then check to see that steam is not too hot. You can either steam over a bowl, making a tent with a towel covering the head, or use a facial sauna bath apparatus. Take care not to steam too long or else dehydration can occur. Steam your face for between 3 and 10 minutes.

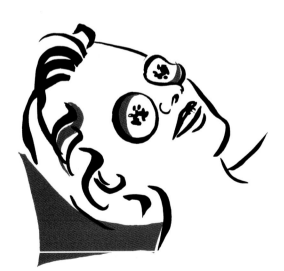

NEXT PAGE:
Fresh living ingredients, found in nature and prepared by you, give the skin and body a wonderful come-alive feeling.

BELOW, EYE TREATMENTS:
Cucumber slices can soothe and brighten tired eyes. See page 33.

tip

Protect sensitive areas of the face as well as the eyes and lips with a protective cream before steaming.

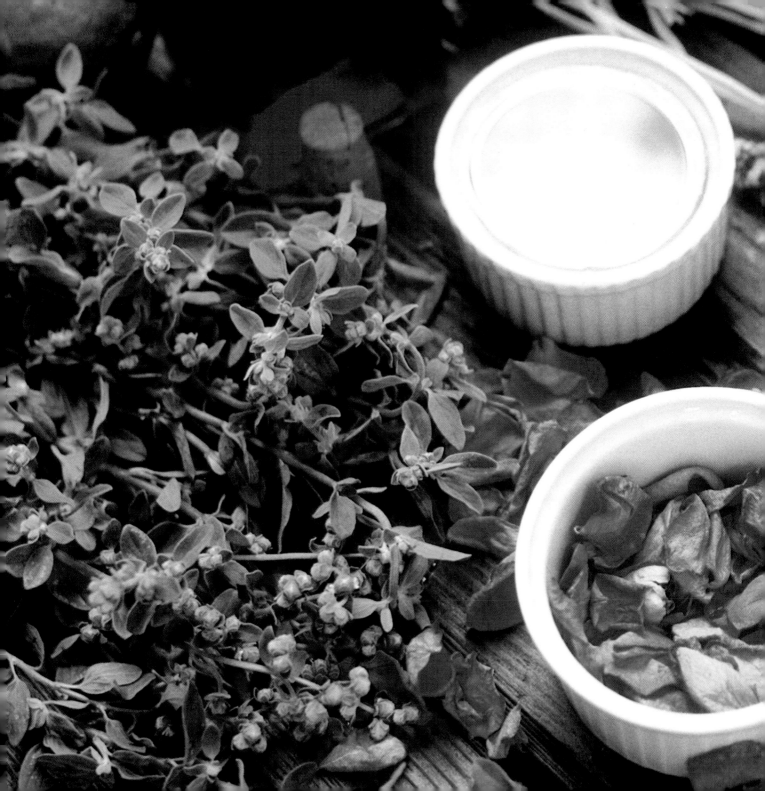

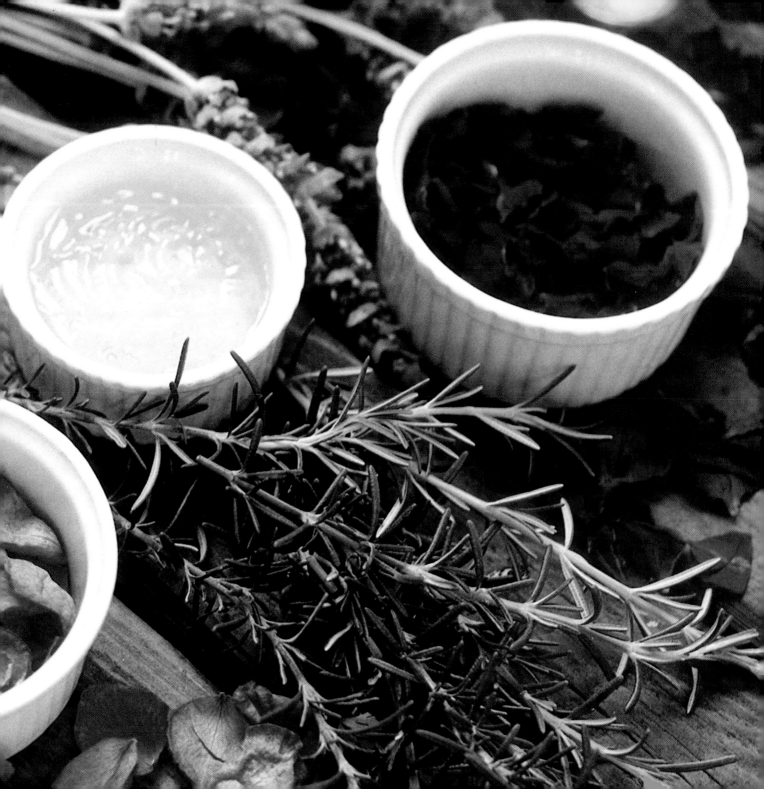

Recipes

Calming pack

If you are unable to sit up, or you have breathing difficulties or a sensitive skin, it is recommended that you use a facial pack.

4 cups fresh camomile
Boiling water to cover

Simmer in pan until leaves combine into a thick mask. Set aside to cool. Spread mask while still warm over a piece of clean muslin (cheesecloth) and apply to your face, avoid the eyes and mouth (cut a hole out for nose and mouth). Leave for 10–15 minutes, then rinse with luke-warm water. Substitute other herbs for camomile to benefit an oily skin condition or perhaps a sensitive acne condition.

Herbal sauna

A stimulating herbal steam bath which will relax and soften the skin.

1 teaspoon dried rosemary
1 teaspoon dried mint leaves
1 teaspoon dried ground fennel seeds
1 teaspoon dried sweet basil
1.75 litres/3 pints/2 quarts boiling water

Mix all the ingredients together and use as above.

The eyes and lips

The eyes

This sensitive area can suffer noticeably from sun, poor diet, allergies, stress overload, fatigue and poor-quality cosmetics. The area of skin around the eyes is thinner because it has fewer oil and perspiration glands to protect it. Always protect your eyes from the drying effects of weather by using eye protective creams and sunglasses. Avoid using sunscreens on the eyes.

To apply an eye cream, bring the cream to body temperature by warming between finger-tips of both hands, pat on gently around the eye. Start from the inner corner of the eye and work outwards. Do not apply directly under the eye as puffiness could occur if ingredients are absorbed into the eyes. Avoid eye creams during the night as there is a chance they may be absorbed into the eyes. Eye fresheners can be used day or night, however, for sore and tired eyes.

There are many eye creams and gels on the market. Go for the waxier ones that are more protective against weather.

The lips

Your lips need protecting too. Lip creams are used for preventing, as well as treating dry, cracked lips. Cold temperatures and exposure to sun and salt water, drying effects of central heating or air conditioning, will cause premature wrinkling around the mouth, appearing as fine lines. Apply lip creams several times a day. Use them under your lipsticks to prevent drying effects of lipsticks. Press lip creams in with fingertips over and around lip line using light pressure to improve circulation.

Recipes

Protective eye cream

Will prevent dryness and premature wrinkling by improving the skin's elasticity. A protective eye cream can prevent and relieve swellings and irritations of the eyelids too.

1 tablespoon beeswax
1 tablespoon cocoa butter (or more if too runny)
1 tablespoon avocado oil
2 teaspoons cod liver oil
2 teaspoons wheatgerm oil
1 tablespoon olive oil or jojoba oil
1 tablespoon almond oil

Melt beeswax and cocoa butter over low heat in a double saucepan (boiler). Remove from heat and mix in all the oils until creamy. Replace the water in double saucepan (boiler) with cold water and stir until cool. Once cool, store in airtight jars.

Eye treatments

TO SOOTHE TIRED EYES – Place a slice of cucumber on each eye for soothing and brightening up the eyes.

TO REDUCE PUFFINESS – Grate 2 slices of peeled raw potato. Place in 2 small pieces of muslin (cheesecloth). Heat 2 teaspoons olive oil to skin temperature and apply to skin around the eyes with dampened cotton wool. Place a potato pad over each eye for 5–10 minutes, rinse with warm water and pat dry.

TO LIGHTEN DARK CIRCLES – Place a slice of apple on each eye for 5–10 minutes.

Relaxation eye mask

Make a rectangular bag out of silk, measuring about 19 x 8.5 cm (7 ½ x 3 ½ inches). Silk will allow skin to breathe and will filter the aromas of herbs more effectively. Fill the bag with finely chopped dried herbs such as lavender, camomile, eyebright. Weigh down, if necessary, with linseed.

Lip saver

1 tablespoon cocoa butter
1 tablespoon beeswax
1 tablespoon avocado oil
2 teaspoons wheatgerm oil
1 tablespoon hydrous lanolin
2 teaspoons olive oil

Melt ingredients over a double saucepan (boiler). Remove and stir. Pour into moulds (old lipstick holders) or jars. They will only take 10 minutes to set. Keep this at room temperature.

Honey lip cream

1 teaspoon clear honey
1 teaspoon melted beeswax
2 teaspoons almond oil

Melt honey and beeswax in a double saucepan (boiler). Add almond oil. Put into a jar and shake well to emulsify. Pour into moulds or jars and allow cream to set for at least 10 minutes before using.

tip

Mother nature has provided us with clay (red, green, yellow, white and pink) and moor (an organic substance formed naturally from over 400 species of herbs and flowers) which have a deep cleansing, toning and restorative action on facial skin and muscles. Applied to the face, they are able to draw tension and toxins away and remove excess acid from the skin – ideal to maintain and enhance your youthful health and beauty without need of a facial massage!

Hair and Nail Care

*H*air and nails are specialized parts of the skin. They contain the protein keratin and are made up of dead cells. The condition of your hair and nails reflects the general health of your body. Many factors, such as weather conditions, seasons, ageing, general and mental health, and changing lifestyle can alter the nutritional requirements of your hair, scalp and nails.

The hair

Hairs are keratinized, dead structures which arise from hair follicles (pore-like indentions in the skin). Each hair follicle has one or more sebaceous glands and a muscle that contracts to make the hair stand on end in response to cold or fright. The chief element of hair follicles is silica, found in all natural foods such as fruits, vegetables and wholegrain cereals. Sebum (oil) from the sebaceous glands is a lubricant for the skin and keeps the hair soft.

The *root* is that portion of the hair that lies inside the *follicle,* the *shaft* is the part of the hair above the skin surface. The base of the root is called the *bulb,* which surrounds a mass of loose connective tissue, the *papilla,* which contains a blood supply and other elements essential for the growth of hair.

On average, hair grows 12 mm/½ inch per month. Each day 25–50 hairs are shed (just as dead surface cells are lost daily from the skin). Once a hair is shed, the follicle degenerates to half its normal length and can take from 60–150 days to reconstruct and begin a new cycle of growth. A normal scalp has between 24 and 40 layers of dead cells which are constantly moving up to the surface where they are shed, and replaced in a 28-day cycle. Dandruff usually means that 20–30 layers are flaking at once, exposing new cells before they are hardened and causing skin sensitivity and damage.

Haircare

Haircare ingredients should be as biologically compatible with skin as possible, and able to work with the natural secretions to provide a nutritional balance. Avoid harsh chemicals and treatments which often contain detergents, thickeners, colours and perfumes as well as toxic substances such as dioxane, formaldehydes, petrochemicals, ethylene oxide and N-nitrosamines, all of which are readily absorbed through the skin. To bring back your hair's essential beauty, natural products are best.

Invest in a natural bristle brush and/or comb to avoid the static electricity produced by plastic. A good, stylish haircut makes using chemical gels and hairsprays unnecessary. It is recommended that your hair is cut every six to eight weeks.

Hair damage

There are many causes of hair damage. You need to protect your hair against over-exposure to hairdryers, heated tongs, perming solutions, chemical hair dyes, chlorinated water and central heating The sun, salt water, hard water and air pollution are also very damaging.

Blow drying can dry out the hair and scalp, so resort to it as little as possible. If your style permits, use only a cool setting and allow the last traces of dampness to evaporate naturally. Never hold the hairdryer in a fixed position. Excessive heat will dry the hair too much and cause damage.

OPPOSITE:
To highlight and beautify the colours of your hair, natural products are best. They are more compatible with the skin because they are free from toxic substances such as petrochemicals, dioxane, formaldehydes, ethylene oxide and N-nitrosamines.

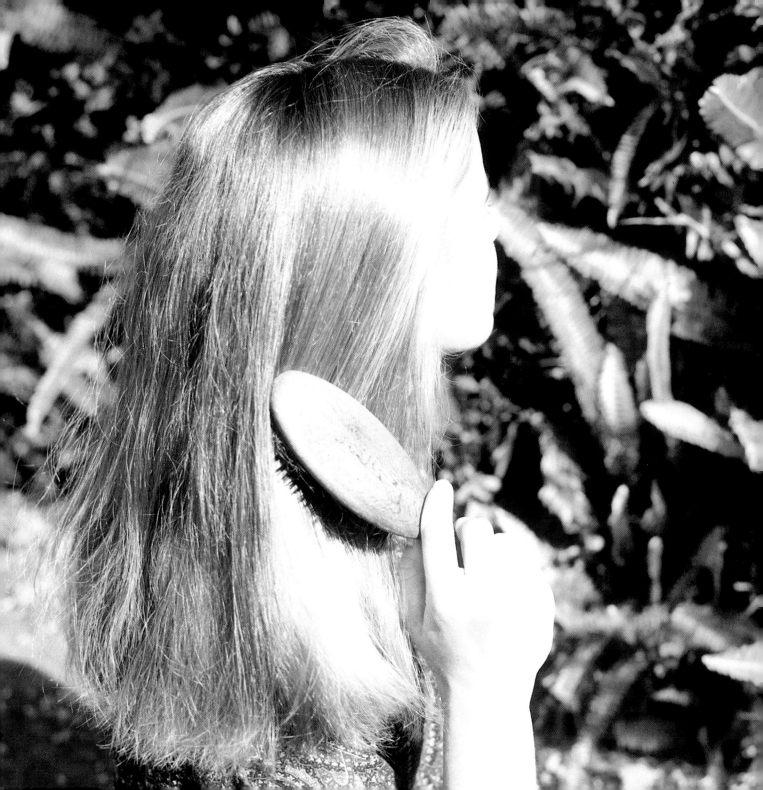

Pre-shampoo treatments

Before applying a pre-shampoo treatment, it is recommended that the hair be free of gels or hairsprays. For dry hair heat a vegetable oil such as apricot kernel oil, or, for normal hair, olive, sesame or jojoba oil until slightly warm. Massage this into the scalp and comb it through. Wrap a hot damp towel around your head and leave for 20 minutes.

These hot oil soakings will soften the scalp and open the pores. Use a strong infusion of camomile tea as a final rinse after shampooing the oil out.

Shampoo

For extra cleanliness and shine, brush your hair before shampooing. The shampoo cleans the hair and opens the pores. Use only a small amount – a lot of lather does not mean the shampoo is more effective. "Squeaky clean" may also indicate that the shampoo has stripped the protective sebum from hair shafts.

Hair rinse/conditioner

A conditioner or hair rinse will close the pores, protecting the hair against the environment and mismanagement. It works as a feeding system for the hair and scalp as well as a detangling agent for easier combing. Stiffness or heaviness of hair may be due to a build-up of 'conditioning' ingredients, which can leave a coating on the hair shaft. Cleanse build-up with a deep-cleansing shampoo and use a lighter conditioner.

Herbs play an important role in keeping hair shiny, strengthening it and stimulating its growth.

tip

If your follicles sit vertically in your scalp, you will have straight hair. If they sit slightly bent, you will have curly hair.

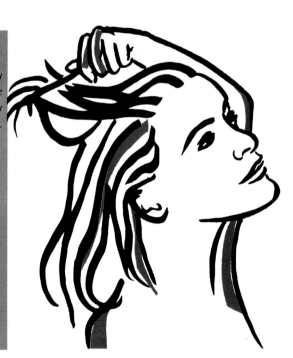

Protein shampoo

This recipe is for brittle, damaged hair. The protein will restore the hair.

3 tablespoons fine wheat flour or pea/bean flour
450 ml/¾ pint/2 cups still mineral or filtered water
1 tablespoon herb vinegar or lemon juice

Mix together and apply mixture slowly to wet scalp and hair.

Honey and oil

1 teaspoon clear honey
3 teaspoons olive oil

Mix and leave to stand for a few hours. Stir well and apply to hair before shampooing. For a final rinse, add a tablespoon of cider vinegar or lemon juice to 1 litre/1¾ pints/4¼ cups pure water.

Egg shampoo

This recipe is to clean the hair and give it a shiny, lighter appearance.

1 or 2 eggs
3 tablespoons still mineral water, warmed
1 tablespoon cider vinegar or lemon juice

Mix the ingredients and apply slowly to wet scalp and hair. Success depends on a long massage and a long rinse under lukewarm water. Use this shampoo straight away as it does not keep. For a final rinse, add a tablespoon of cider vinegar or lemon juice to the water for shine and body.

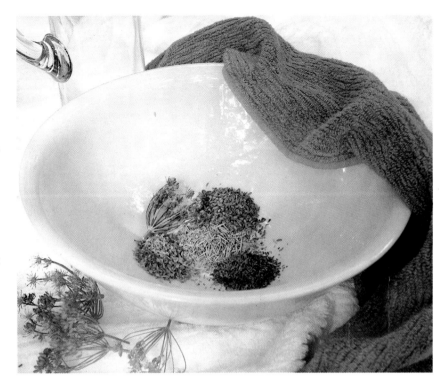

Steeping fresh herbs

Herbs for hair need to steep for as long as 2–3 hours. Make a herbal infusion by pouring boiling water (600 ml/1 pint/2½ cups) over fresh or dried herbs. Dried herbs will last longer in the refrigerator – perhaps 1 week. After shampooing, use the infusions by using a catch bowl and pouring liquid over your hair several times, against gravity.

Combine or use as a single hair rinse, sage, parsley and rosemary – gives dark hair a sheen; rosemary is excellent for controlling colours.

Combine camomile, calendula and yarrow flowers for highlighting blond, dark or mousy coloured hair.

ABOVE:
A herbal infusion makes a wonderful hair rinse after shampooing. See the Steeping fresh herbs recipe opposite.

OPPOSITE:

To prevent dry nails and cuticles,
soak your fingertips in a warm oil
bath for 5-10 minutes.

Dry shampoo

Sprinkle a handful of bran or oatmeal through hair, gently massage scalp and hair for a few minutes. Brush out.

Handy rinses and conditioners

LEMON RINSE – 2 teaspoons lemon juice to a bowl of water encourages the hair shaft to lie hair in the right direction. Will also lighten hair, even dark hair, in sun.

CIDER VINEGAR RINSE – Use 125 ml/4 fl oz/½ cup cider vinegar to every 1 litre/1¾ pints/4¼ cups water. Will promote shine.

BEER RINSE – A homemade brew is excellent for conditioning the hair and adding shine. Can make dark hair lighter in the sun.

RAIN WATER – Filter it, boil it up and mix with a herb to steep. Rain water will give hair extra softness.

COCONUT OIL – Gives your hair a lovely shine and protects against the elements. Apply before swimming and sunbathing.

Hair spray

1 lemon (oily hair) or 1 orange (dry hair)
450 ml/3/4 pint/2 cups water

Chop up fruit, add to water in saucepan and simmer until reduced by half. Strain and put into a spray gun.

The nails

The condition of your nails reflects the general health of your body. The nail is whitish in appearance, allowing the healthy pink of the nail bed to be seen. Nails are an appendage of the skin and they protect the tips of the fingers and toes.

The *nail root* is at the base of the nail, underneath the skin and covered by the cuticle. It originates from the *matrix* which is the part of the nail bed that produces the new nail as new cells form and harden. The matrix contains nerves, and blood and lymph vessels and it determines the character, health and strength of the nail. The pearly half-moon, or *lunula,* is the only visible section of the matrix.

The *nail bed* is a continuation of the matrix and is supplied with blood vessels necessary to nourish the growing nail. The *nail plate* is the part of the visible nail that rests upon and is attached to the nail bed. Its scaly dead-cell layers are held together with a small amount of moisture and fat. The *free edge* is the whitish part of the nail extending beyond the nail plate.

The *nail walls* are folds of skin overlapping the sides of the nail. Like all skin, the nail walls constantly produce new cells and cast off old ones. The *cuticle* is the overlapping epidermis around the nail.

Nail care

CLEANING – Use a pure bristle nail brush. Use an orange stick to clean underneath nails too.
CUTICLE TREATMENT – Use an oil or nail cream and massage around the cuticle with a firm rotary movement, using cushion of thumbs. Finish off by tapering the tips of each finger with an upward movement. Leave oil or cream on for 10–20 minutes and, with an orange stick, gently lift cuticle along each side of the nail (not the base) without scraping nail. Wrap cotton cloth around each finger and wipe

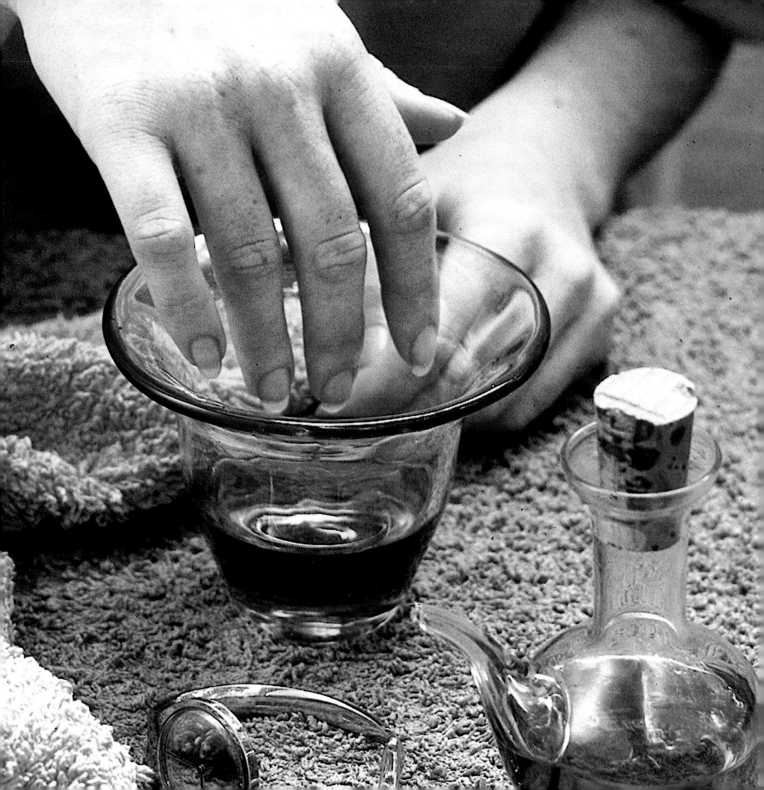

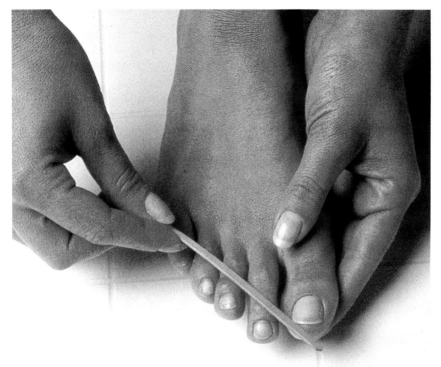

away dead cuticle from each nail, gently pushing back cuticle in the process. Use cuticle clippers to trim loose pieces of cuticle from the sides, but never around the base.

SHAPING – File carefully from side to centre, then from the other side to centre with the coarse side of the emery board, shaping the nails square to tip of finger (this protects the nail) then shape the oval. Nails will appear longer and wear better if you allow the sides of the nails to grow. Do not file deep into the corners of the nail or you weaken the free edge, exposing the nail to splitting and cracking.

BUFFING – increases circulation in the fingertips, smooths nails and gives a natural gloss. Buff nails with downward strokes – from the base down to the free edge.

Special nail treatments

BRITTLE NAILS – Drink 3 teaspoons of gelatine dissolved in fruit juice each morning. Eating a balanced diet will benefit the health of skin, hair and nails.

RIDGED NAILS – Try an oil manicure. Warm up vegetable (preferably olive) oil and soak fingers for 5–10 minutes. Massage hands and wrists with warm oil too. Remove oil with a warm, damp towel. Also good for preventing dryness of nails and cuticles and for softening hands.

ABOVE:

The only difference between toenail and fingernail care, is that toenails should never be shaped. Trim toenails straight across the top of the toe – do not shape. Use a file to smooth the cut edge.

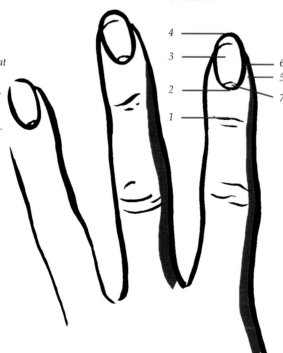

STRUCTURE OF THE NAIL:

1   Matrix
2   Nail root
3   Nail plate
4   Free edge
5   Nail bed
6   Cuticle
7   Lunula

Recipes

Nail-biters' aid

Nail-biting, often caused by nervous tension, can be improved with the use of these calming essential oils. You can leave this oil on to soften and protect the cuticles, too.

1 drop camomile essential oil
1 drop lavender essential oil
1 teaspoon vegetable oil, for example olive, almond or grapeseed

Combine ingredients and gently massage cuticles (see Cuticle treatment, page 38).

Pineapple cuticle cream

This recipe is to soften the cuticles.

1 tablespoon pineapple juice
1 tablespoon egg yolk
¼ teaspoon cider vinegar

Combine the ingredients and soak the nails for 30 minutes. Rinse.

Avocado nail cream

Mash a small portion of avocado and massage into cuticles and nails. Very nourishing.

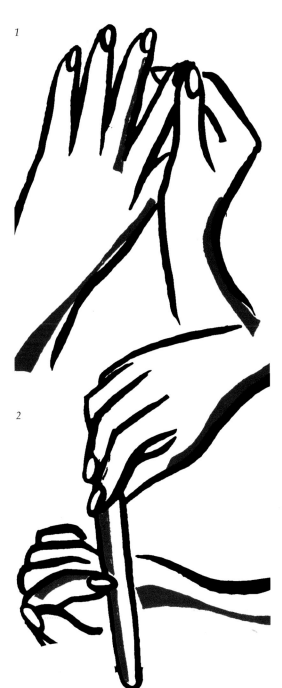

NAIL CARE:
1   Massage oil into the cuticles
2   File the nails

Looking Good

Make-up is a wonderful way of enhancing your natural beauty and character, making the most of your best features. Applying make-up is an art form – a creative expression of your individuality. Also clothes look more stylish when complemented by good make-up that is applied well.

Wear the colours that suit your skin's undertones to gain confidence as your true colours shine through. Using colours that are not complementary to your skin's unique undertone colourings can give you an unnatural appearance, and make you feel as if you are hiding behind a mask.

Make-up will always appear more radiant if your skin is clean and healthy. Less make-up will be required too. However, even with a blemished skin, heavy make-up is not necessarily needed these days, with the availability of concealers. It is better to camouflage than to wear heavier make-up, especially during the day. A natural, lighter look is always more complementary as well as more comfortable to wear.

There is an increasing number of quality, natural make-up ranges available from health food shops and some department stores. They prefer to use ingredients that are of natural origin such as beeswax, vegetable oils, earth minerals and plant pigments. Look for unscented products that are also free from petrochemical derivatives.

Have fun experimenting with make-up and the different ways of applying it. Do not be afraid to use the testers on shop counters. Make-up consultants can also provide helpful ideas and answers, or a full personal analysis if you wish. There is a wide selection of make-up from which to choose, so it is worthwhile shopping around until you find what you feel comfortable with.

OPPOSITE:
Many natural make-up ranges are becoming available from health shops and department stores. Natural make-up uses no harmful ingredients, such as petro-chemicals and colours, and is not tested on animals.

Skin undertones

Everyone has unique colour tonings. Your skin tone is a blend of three pigments, melanin (brown), carotene (yellow) and haemoglobin (red), and your colourings are either warm or cool. Looking into a mirror during daylight without any make-up on, will give you an indication of your undertone. You will also see the undertones on your wrist and hands against white paper, which is more accurate. Your skin type will fit into one of the four basic undertones groups that are described below.

Warm undertones

GOLDEN YELLOW/ORANGE UNDERTONES – These skin types range from palest ivory, peaches and cream, to golden creamy yellow, through to dark olive and yellow-black. These skin colourings suit delicate colours and tones such as coral, warm pink, peach, grey-brown (taupe for example), mushroom, cocoa, smoked mauve and plum.

PEACHY RED/ORANGE UNDERTONES – These skin types range from fair ivory or peach with freckles, to golden beige, peachy pink and ruddy, through to golden brown, copper and coppery/black. These skin colourings suit rich autumn tones such as orange, russet, ginger, tawny pink and golden brown.

Cool undertones

PINK UNDERTONES – These skin types range from very pale or white (with little or no melanin), to brown and rosy-beige, through to olive and black (with a

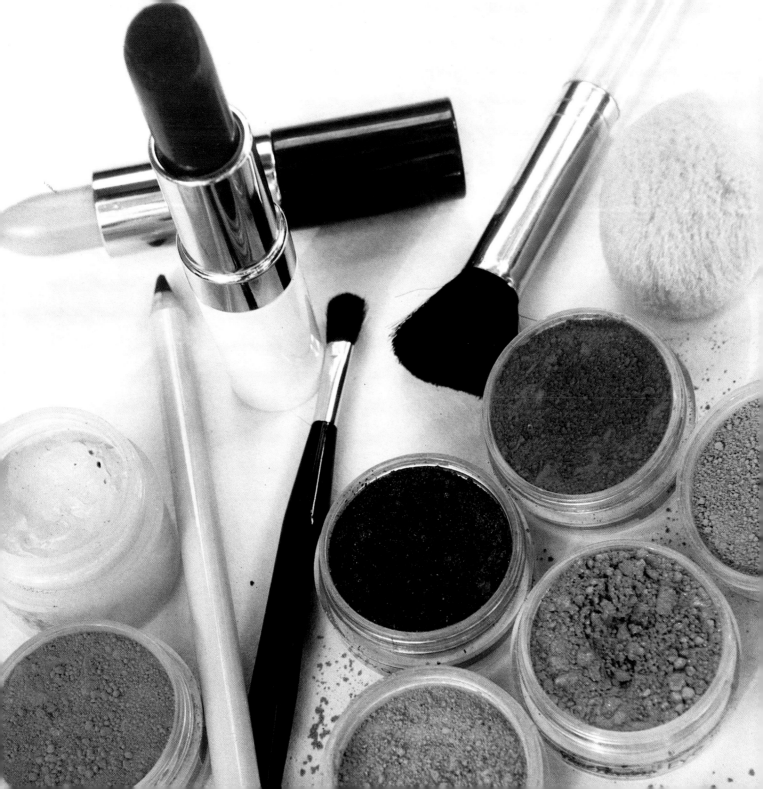

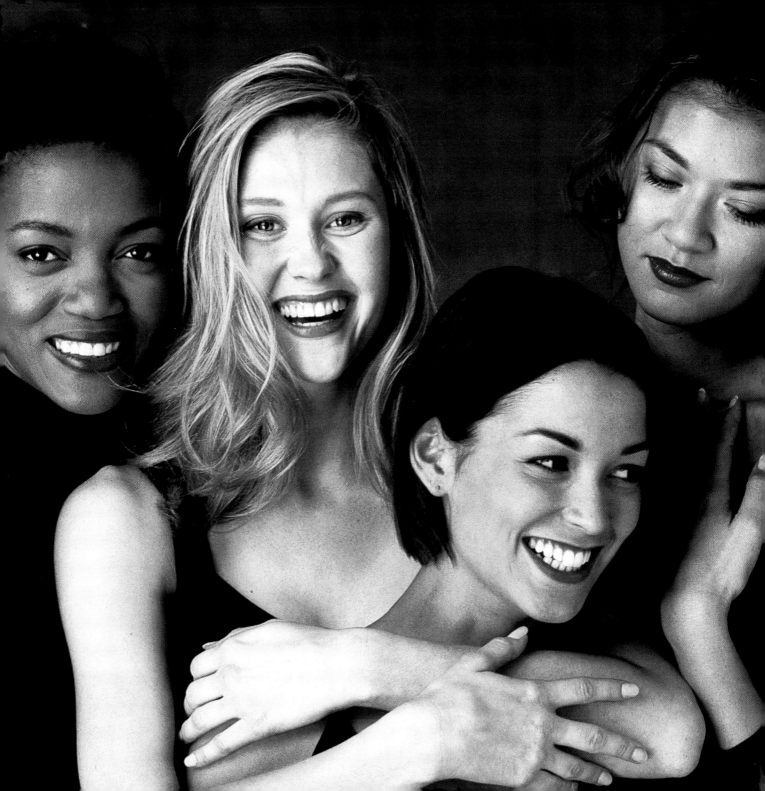

lot of melanin). These skin colourings suit either vivid primary colours or very cool colours.

BLUE/PINK UNDERTONES – These skin types range from translucent, sand, pale beige with delicate pink cheeks or no cheek colour, through to rosy pink, rosy brown or grey/purple/brown. These skin colourings suit natural tones such as soft blue and pastel shades.

Complementary make-up

Your skin undertones need to be taken into consideration in the choice of make-up. Colours and tones chosen to complement your undertones will enhance your natural beauty and make the most of your features.

Adapt your choice of colour and tone to suit the occasion and the seasons. There are three facets to consider when applying make-up – undertone, depth and clarity. These factors will determine the over-all look of the make-up. For example, use bold make-up with a bold dress style and softer make-up with a softer, flowing style.

UNDERTONE – Your skin undertone will determine whether you should apply a warm or a cool 'base tone'. If you have a blue/pink undertone, for example, apply a cool 'base tone'.

DEPTH – The darkness or lightness of a tone. The depth of a tone is determined by the amount of black or white added. An example of a dark tone is maroon (black added), and a light tone is pink (white added).

CLARITY – The brightness or softness of a tone. Each colour has its own clarity, that ranges from bright to soft. For example, grey can be added to a colour to achieve a soft tone.

Applying make-up

To get the best from your make-up it should be applied in the following order:

Concealers

Concealers are used before applying foundation. They come in tubes and sticks of light, medium and dark shades and will cover blemishes, spots, high cheek colour, dark circles under the eyes. Lightly dot on with brush or cotton bud and press on with sponge, which will avoid blending around the eyes which may drag the skin. Best applied under a liquid foundation which will conceal naturally.

Foundation

As the name suggests, foundation provides a secure and even surface to which make-up can easily adhere. It will give your skin an even tone, neutralizing red cheeks, freckles and veins. It is not used to change your colour. Foundation is either light, medium or dark, depending on your skin shade. Note that skin shades may change – your slight summer tan may require a darker shade. A shade can be chosen confidently once your skin undertone is determined. Test appropriate shades within your undertone range by applying small amounts each of light, medium and dark on to your jawline or forehead.

When you have found your correct shade, choose between a liquid base foundation and an oily base foundation. Liquid base is lighter to wear, suitable for daytime use and used on oily skin or younger skin that does not require much coverage. Oily base is more appropriate for covering up and camouflaging, as well as for night use. It is more flattering under lighting and is recommended for use on stage or for special photographs such as wedding pictures where features need to stand out better.

OPPOSITE:
Everybody has unique skin undertones (see Skin undertones, page 42). Enhance your natural beauty and make the most of your features, by applying colours and tones that complement your skin undertones.

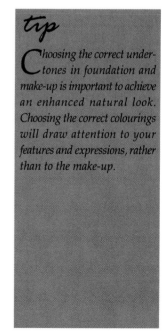

tip

Choosing the correct undertones in foundation and make-up is important to achieve an enhanced natural look. Choosing the correct colourings will draw attention to your features and expressions, rather than to the make-up.

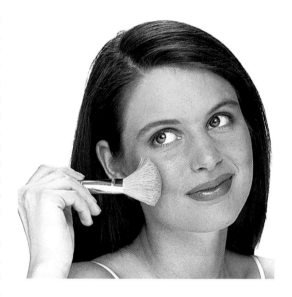

BLENDING – is the secret of even coverage. Use the back of your hand as a palette and blend with fingertips or a moist natural sponge. Apply all over the face, more lightly around the eyes where it may accentuate wrinkles. If too heavy, foundation will stick to dry patches and blemishes. Spread foundation to about 12 mm/½ inch from hairline and use sides of hands to spread over to the hairline. Use downward movement to settle fine downy hair, but take care as you can easily over-stretch muscles. Fade the foundation away to nothing on the throat. Check your foundation coverage in natural light to make sure no major differences are seen between the face and neck.

COLOURED SKIN – FOUNDATION – There is a wide range of foundation shades to suit dark brown, brown, yellow and red skin tones. Dark brown skin foundation is richer in colour but more transparent, less oily than usual because of tendency for darker skin to be drier. Because of the pigmentation, sometimes a translucent powder alone over a moisture base will give an effective natural skintone look. Use only a light application of powder, otherwise skin can turn greyish and look too obvious.

SHADING OR CONTOURING WITH FOUNDATION – Use a combination of two foundations, one light and one dark (both matching the skin undertone, otherwise you will only notice colour and not the face), to disguise features such as a bent nose or large jaw, that can make people feel a little self-conscious. The basic rule for shading is to use the light shades for enhancing features and the darker shades for reducing the emphasis of the imperfection. Set with powder. This technique is less noticeable used at night.

Powders

They are applied after foundation to take away shine and set the make-up. Translucent powders, rather than coloured powders, should be used over your foundation. A natural look will come from the foundation's undertones rather than the colour of powders.

LOOSE POWDERS – are best used over oily-base foundation, otherwise make-up can appear too thick. Use on oily skin conditions for absorbing excess oil to take away a shiny film. Loose powders are not recommended for dry skin as they tend to show up dryness too much.

COMPACT FOUNDATIONS OR BLOCK POWDERS – Use over a liquid base foundation or, better still, on their own. For a matt look, apply block powder to the face with a wet or dry sponge. For a sheer look, dust on with a brush.

Blushers

Blushers enliven the face with the warmth of natural skin tonings. Blusher can be used, like foundation, for shading or contouring your features.

POWDER BLUSHERS – To apply, load a large brush with blusher colour, blow on it to remove any excess

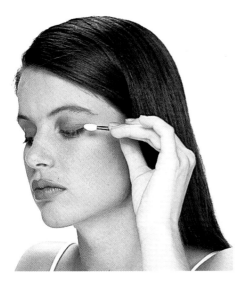

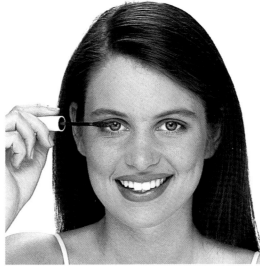

FAR LEFT:

Choose eyeshadow shades and highlighters to complement your skin undertones. Apply the colour with a small brush. Smudge it upwards, towards the brow, fading it away.

LEFT:

Apply mascara to the bottom lashes first. Then apply to the upper lashes using upward strokes.

blush and fluff it lightly on over the cheekbones. Start at hairline and work short strokes down to no further than outer corner of your eye and no lower than the end of your nose. Avoid circle area of your eyes and blend edges for a natural look.

Eyebrow pencils

Eyebrow pencils can change the thickness and shape of brows to balance your overall make-up look. When applying eyebrow pencils, hold the pencil between the thumb and first finger towards the unsharpened end to prevent creating a hard, false line by using too much pressure. Try using two or three different pencils for a natural look as the brows are made up of hairs of many colours.

Eyeshadows

The eyes are the most expressive and beautiful part of the face. The mirror to the soul.

Eyeshadows are easier to use than crayons on most eyes, but do not get any in your eyes. If you prefer crayons, ensure they are creamy and will not stretch the skin around the eyes.

Choose three or four colours, keeping them within the same skin undertone range. Different colours alter length, width, shape and perspective of a face, just as much as they affect dimensions of a room. Always aim for a softer look during the day as there is less contrast of colour than at night when you can apply darker and more exotic colours a little more heavily.

Try different methods of application until you find a look you like. Choosing shades and highlighters in the brown, beige and cream coloured ranges gives a good natural look on a younger face. Older faces suit a light application of eyeshadow. Try colours such as light and dark blues, greys and greens to achieve a natural look.

Sometimes, just one colour will work. Smudge it upwards towards the brow fading it away. Apply thinly to lower lid under the lashes. Use a natural lip colour or gloss to balance the natural look.

tip

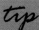

Never reshape your natural eyebrow line as it frames your eyes. Only pluck eyebrows from underneath the line, taking care to support the skin by holding firmly. Pluck in the direction of hair growth to ensure regrowth occurs evenly. You can brush your eyebrows upwards towards the forehead to achieve a softer look using an eyebrow brush.

tip

Maintain your brushes and sponges by regularly cleaning with hot, soapy water and drying in sunlight. When drying, make sure the brush hairs are together rather than fan shaped. This will prevent messy make-up especially with eye brushes and lip brushes.

Eyeliners

Pencil eyeliners are less messy and safer to use than liquid ones. Coordinated with eye-shadows, they can create many different illusions to make eyes appear wider, small, large or open, etcetera.

Darker eye pencils, particularly black, like the Indian kohl, will accentuate the whites of eyes. Thicker kohl was said to protect the eyes. Apply before eyeshadows or just after a base eyeshadow to create a blended, muted look. Fade the line away on outer edge so there is no abrupt end. A sharper, heavier outline can give you a more dramatic look. Apply liquid eyeliner after eyeshadow.

Mascaras

Mascaras are used for thickening and lengthening eyelashes and to tone eyeshadow on lid down. Use the basic shades of black, brown and blue during the day and other colours such as greens, greys, plums are better used for evenings when the lighting can enrich the colour.

To apply mascara, work close to the mirror, start with bottom lashes, longer lashes first. Apply with upward strokes to upper lashes and then use the tip of a wand at the corners of the eyes.

Lipliners/pencils

These are applied around the outline of the lips to prevent lipstick from feathering and can change or enhance the shape of the lips.

Lipliner will stay on longer and will give shape to lips, even when lipstick has worn off. Lipliners are slightly darker in colour than your lipstick. To apply, begin at the centre of the lips and work outwards, to one side then the other.

Lipsticks and lip glosses

Lipsticks tend to be bought and worn more liberally and are available in sticks or pots, matt and frosted. Lipsticks can harmonize make-up by complementing the tonings used on the eyes.

To apply, outline lips first with a lip brush, then begin your application at the centre of the lips and work outwards to the left, then to the right. If your application is in one straight line it will make the lipstick crooked.

Frosted lipsticks will need blotting. Blot the lipstick with a tissue between your lips, hold it over the lips and dust with loose powder before applying a second coat. This makes the lipstick last longer. To add some shine, apply a lip gloss over the top.

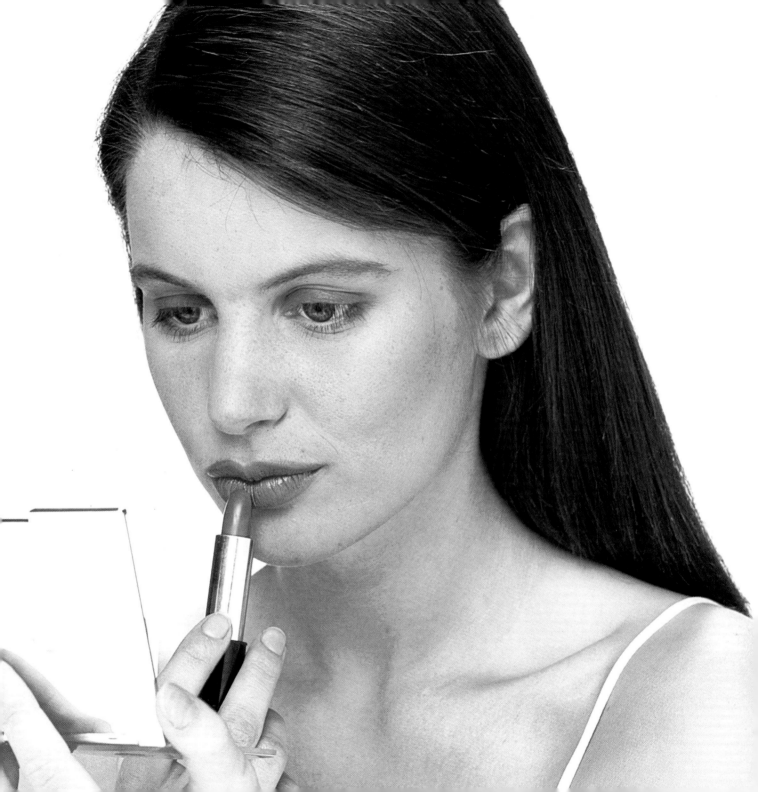

Protecting your Skin

We need to protect the face and body from all harmful effects of the environment, especially from the sun. The worsening depletion of the ozone layer (caused by fluorocarbon propellants in aerosols and the emission of high-flying aircraft) means that we have to protect ourselves more conscientiously than ever before.

Our immune systems are being bombarded every day by artificial additives, preservatives, colourings and other harmful ingredients in food we eat and the cosmetics we apply to the skin. We are also exposed to increasing pollution in the earth's atmosphere which we are breathing into our bodies. The skin, in particular the horny layer and the epidermis, acts as our protection from these harmful influences. Once these top layers of skin tissue have been damaged, the underlying dermis is exposed, allowing all the harmful influences to gain ready access to the rest of the body through its vascular and lymphatic systems.

Skin needs to be nurtured and encouraged to regenerate so it will protect the body to its full capacity. To ensure that regeneration can continually occur, cosmetics should come from nature and be akin to the skin. When people resort to substitution therapy rather than support therapy (see page 13), the skin's natural defences cannot operate effectively to protect the body. As the skin comes to rely on artificial products, it becomes weak and sensitive. Genuinely natural cosmetics do not place such heavy burdens on the skin, allowing it to function more efficiently and promoting a healthier relationship between the skin and the body.

The sun and your skin

The sun is essential to our survival. It is also a natural antibiotic. The sun also has an influence over substances in the skin called sterols, which convert to vitamin D, enabling calcium to be absorbed in the body. Only small amounts are required by the body at any one time for health and well-being.

The sun is the main cause of skin ageing, apart from the process of growing old. Sun causes moisture loss in the skin almost as soon as we are exposed to it after childbirth. The majority of damage caused by the sun is usually realized during childhood. Following are three types of harmful ultraviolet (UV) rays:

UVA (LONGER TANNING RAYS) – connected with the ageing process.
UVB (SHORTER BURNING RAYS) – potentially the most dangerous and cause of most skin cancers.
UVC RAYS – absorbed by earth's atmosphere, but linked to eye damage.

UV rays cause the formation of substances called 'free radicals' which damage the DNA and the connective tissue of the skin. The damage caused can lie dormant for 30 years or more but can result in a weakening of the immune system, leading to a variety of skin cancers. Other harmless rays include visible light and infra-red heat.

OPPOSITE:
You can still enjoy the benefits of the sun if you take proper care to protect yourself against the damaging effects of ultraviolet radiation.

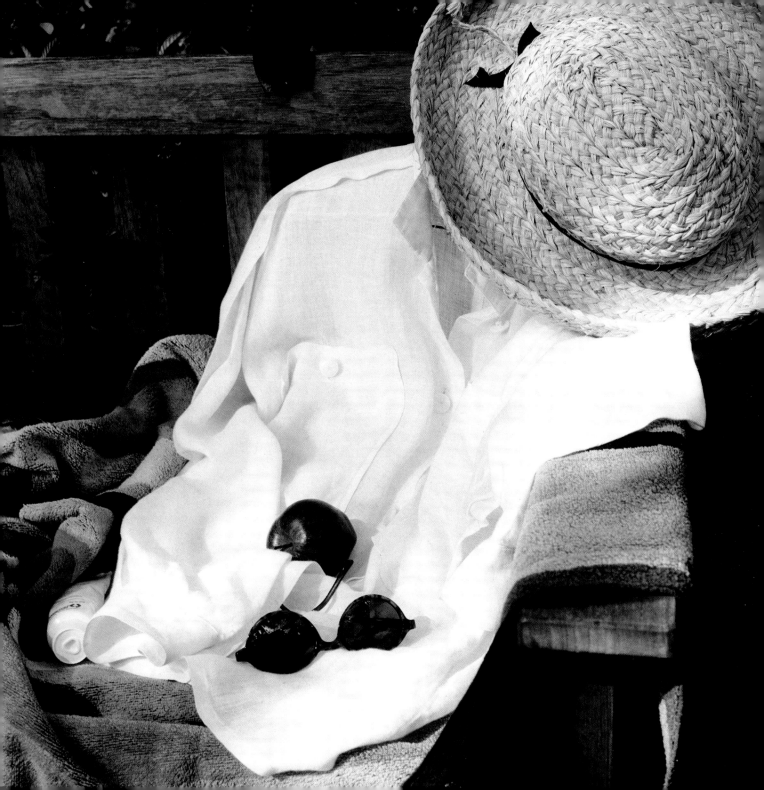

The sun is stronger closer to the Equator and sun damage is greater as the sun's rays hit the earth at right angles and are less filtered by the atmosphere. Damage can affect all skin types, regardless of racial background, colour or occupation. Dark brown skin is naturally protected as melanin is produced faster and this skin type will cool faster. Dark brown skin also has more sweat and sebaceous glands to provide a protective film. Some people will be more susceptible to sun damage, such as redheads, who freckle easily and who have fewer melanocytes.

Causes of skin damage

Skin damage does not always happen in the sun at the beach. Water, sand, snow and cement reflect the sun's rays. Ultraviolet rays injure living cells and lower the body's immune system by penetrating the skin and causing these cells to swell up and the skin to burn.

Damage will accumulate tan after tan. It takes only 10 minutes for an average skin to burn. If you eat a sensible diet, rich in vitamins and minerals from fresh living foods (that are as free from chemicals as possible), you will reduce the risk of abnormal skin conditions and reactions. A heavy consumption of meat and starch in the diet can make the skin prone to skin cancer.

Abusive cleansing techniques, such as the use of peels and scrubs, can damage the protective horny layer and in turn the epidermis, leaving the body unprotected and exposed fully to the elements and to harmful and artificially prepared ingredients in cosmetics.

Artificial sweeteners and some medicines can make the skin sensitive to light or can be harmful to take when exposing yourself to sun. They include antibiotics, oral contraceptives, sulphur drugs, diuretics, cortisones, antihistamines, tranquillizers, vegetable-based laxatives. Some essential oils can also cause sensitivity in strong sunlight. Perfumes and aftershaves (which are mixtures of pure or synthetic essential oils) can all leave their mark, being highly photosensitive as well.

Skin's natural defences

When the skin is well maintained it will more easily defend the body against different environments and enable us to adapt to changing environmental conditions.

Melanin is the dark pigment that protects the skin from too much sun. Melanocytes are produced in the first few hours of sun exposure, tanning skin straight away as a protection against further injury. Other melanin granules are transferred to the skin cells two to three days after bathing in the sun.

The colour will fade only when the melanin in the lower layers of the skin gradually rises to the skin surface during the regeneration process. Raw vegetables help the skin produce plenty of melanin.

New skin cells can form at a faster rate, if need be, providing a new, thicker skin to act as a barricade against the wind. A leathery skin appearance may result, however.

Sun protection

The face, in particular, is exposed to the elements all the year round. Be aware that too much sunshine can be dangerous.

Keep exposure to the sun at an absolute minimum. In very sunny conditions avoid the sun between the hours of 11am and 3pm when it is at its strongest and – most importantly – always cover up. Wear a wide-brimmed hat to protect the scalp and face, and sunglasses that have 99 per cent protection from UV rays and polarizing lenses to cut down the reflected glare. The glasses should also be of a close-fitting, wrap-around style. These are available for children too.

Loose cotton clothing offers the best protection from UV light. The Arabs had the right idea in adopting maximum protection with a burnoose or djellaba. Middle Eastern cultures keep the body and head fully covered with cotton clothing and wear veils over the face. The return of long dresses, gloves, hats and umbrellas would not be such a bad idea!

Sunscreens

Chemical sunscreens are very important for protecting the skin against UV rays. They act by selectively blocking out the wavelengths of light that cause UV damage to your complexion.

There are many sunscreen ingredients, but there are only two recommended sunscreens at present – cinnamate (absorbs light) and titanium (deflects light). Both protect the body from UVA and UVB rays. Titanium is recommended for children under 12 months. (Babies should not be exposed to the sun at all.) Cinnamate will be absorbed by the skin and is a more readily available sunscreen.

Chemical sunscreens have been used successfully for protecting the skin from harmful UV rays for the last 10 years. However, not enough research has been done into their long-term effects or into the effects they have when combined with other ingredients. When buying sunscreens, look at the labels and avoid those with a lengthy list of ingredients.

What to look for

It is always best to choose a maximum protection, broad spectrum sunscreen with a Sun Protection Factor (SPF) of 15+. This offers the highest form of chemical sunscreen protection against UVA and UVB rays (94 per cent). Always make sure that it is water resistant, especially if you are going to the beach, so that you will not have to reapply your sunscreen more often than the SPF recommendation.

Apply sunscreen cream, oil, milk or gel 10 to 15 minutes before going outdoors to enable it to be absorbed and bonded to the skin. Determine the length of time the sunscreen will protect you by multiplying the SPF by 10 minutes, for example 15x10 minutes = 150 minutes of protection. The range of sunscreens available include:

MAXIMUM PROTECTION – SPF 15+
HIGH PROTECTION – SPF 8–14
MODERATE PROTECTION – SPF 4–7
MINIMUM PROTECTION – SPF 2–3

Other factors

Sunburn is intensified by wind. Your skin is at even greater risk during outdoor activities such as skiing or mountain climbing because there is less atmosphere at high altitude to absorb the sun's rays. Your skin may become sensitive and irritable after exposure to the sun, wind or cold as moisture depletion causes dryness and chapping. There are seasonal variations too. During hot summer months you will notice your skin perspiring and becoming slightly more oily. In the cooler seasons skin tends to dry out in heated air inside your home and in cold, dry air outside. (See Moisturizers pages 18,22,24.)

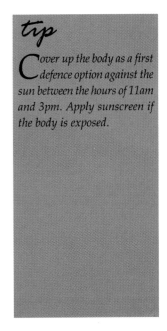

tip

Cover up the body as a first defence option against the sun between the hours of 11am and 3pm. Apply sunscreen if the body is exposed.

Responding to Skin Condition

Skin undergoes so many changes, because of weather, sickness, allergy, pregnancy, puberty and menopause, it is sometimes difficult to recognize a particular condition. Once you can determine the condition of the skin, however, appropriate steps can be taken to encourage the skin to normalize.

Normal skin

Normal skin is smooth and moist with a healthy glow. Do not take normal skin for granted. Always maintain healthy skin by proper cleansing, adequate protection, a balanced diet and plenty of water, sleep and relaxation.

Dry skin

Dry skin will have a parched or scaly appearance with no obvious sebaceous gland opening. It lacks oil and it is fragile. There will be a tendency to develop premature wrinkles if it is not carefully looked after.

CAUSES – Dryness occurs when the outer part of the skin loses moisture at too rapid a rate. It is the body struggling to keep up with the conditions the skin is exposed to. A lack of elasticity due to the loss of water in the skin will promote oils in the skin to become clogged, causing blackheads for example.

TREATMENT – Skin oils are unsaturated and appear to be made almost completely of essential fatty acids, similar to vegetable oils. Including vegetable oils in your diet will benefit this skin condition. Foods containing silica will enable the connective tissue to strengthen also. To soften skin and prevent moisture loss, use oil-based protective creams.

Oily skin

Oily skin is caused by the overproduction of oil which can clog the skin causing blemishes, blackheads, whiteheads, pimples and acne. Sometimes there is also a flaky appearance caused by the accumulation of dried-out oils from the skin. The skin will almost always have a shiny film with larger pores.

CAUSES – A reactive oily skin condition (reactive seborrhoea), will have an abnormal amount of oil coming from the sebaceous glands from over-stimulation of the skin, sometimes from washing too much. Moisture loss and sweat will signal the oil glands to take over.

TREATMENT – Deep cleansing is necessary twice a day. Soak the skin using the antitoxic and antiseptic properties of essential oils such as lemon, bergamot, geranium, juniper or lavender to prevent and clear congestion in the skin. Applying light vegetable oils to the oily surface for protection will enable the excess oils in the skin to flow out on to the skin, rather than becoming clogged in dry pores.

Treat the oiliness with oil, until skin starts to show improvement, then start to use a light moisturizer. Avoid excess shine on the face by dusting lightly with powder to absorb oils, or blot the skin with a tissue.

Sensitive skin

Sensitive skin is usually a combination of conditions. It can be red or pink in appearance and often shows a tendency towards broken capillaries and dryness. Quite often the skin is congested and acidic. The skin surface is usually without defences, allowing weather damage to deeper skin layers. It can also react allergically from application of different products and can be a sign that the body is also sensitive.

TREATMENT – Work from within to strengthen and

OPPOSITE:

Many beautiful bottles that can be used to store your vegetable and essential oil mixtures are available. The glass stoppers can be used to apply lotion (see page 17). Coloured glass also enables homemade preparations to have a longer shelf life.

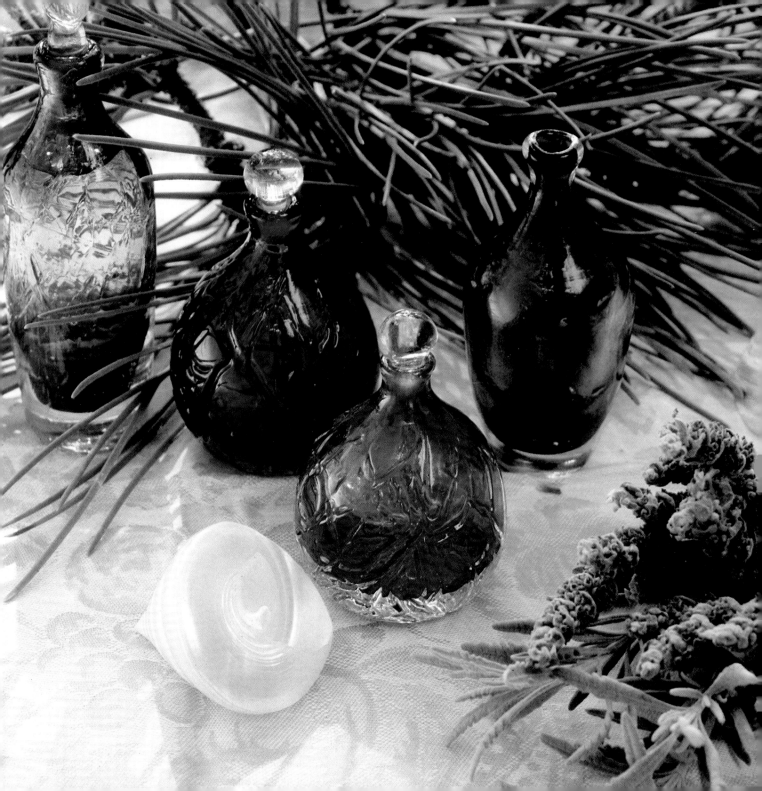

cleanse the organs to improve circulation of blood and lymph. The body needs a balanced diet and lifestyle. Make sure you use protective creams during treatment. Sensitive skin will fluctuate from one extreme of oiliness (acid) to extremes of dryness (alkaline). Skin needs a balance of oil and water.

Dehydrated skin

Dehydrated skin lacks water, and will quickly become wrinkled. Once it has lost elasticity, the skin's subcutaneous layer may become saggy, and the face will appear drawn.

CAUSES – The person is usually dehydrated and thin with a tendency towards endocrine imbalance or low kidney energy. Often cold.

TREATMENT – Rehydrate the body and organs by drinking water and avoiding the stimulants that can be very dehydrating. Essential oil therapy can also be useful. For warmth, use olive oil – apply to the skin, massage in as well, or add to bath.

Hydrated skin

People with hydrated skin have excess water and sweat easily. Their skin is very sensitive to the surrounding atmospheric conditions.

CAUSE – Excess water loss from the skin indicates an overconsumption of fluids, overburdened kidneys or an overworked heart.

Watery skin

People with watery skin suffer from water retention that can have a puffy appearance.

CAUSE – Mainly congestion due to a spleen or lymphatic condition. You may be doing too much and working your adrenals overtime!

TREATMENT – Relaxation can enable the body to improve circulation, benefiting a sluggish lymph system (see Understanding Your Skin, page 8).

Acne

Acne is an inflammation of the hair follicles, preceded by an increase of fatty discharges. The ducts of the sebaceous glands become clogged and the skin becomes greasy with appearance of skin impurities. A small abscess results after inflamed follicles fuse together. Pock marks can be left after abscesses heal. Acne can affect the face, chest and back and the skin can be extremely painful to touch at times. Acne sufferers may experience a combination of skin ailments such as oiliness, dryness, infection, sensitivity, allergies and inflammation.

People with acne, especially teenagers, can become very self-conscious and lose their self-esteem. Acne can start as early as 12 to 14 years but diminishes in severity by 18 to 20 years, usually disappearing by the age of 25 to 30.

CAUSES – Oil glands are inactive in childhood and develop at puberty. Common acne is a result of a disorder of the skin's metabolism, which is closely linked with the physical and psychological changes of puberty.

TREATMENT – There is no known cure for acne, but it can be treated most successfully by keeping the disease under control until it clears with time. The system can be cleansed by a diet free of refined sugars, preservatives and artificial colours – tending more towards a vegetarian and low-fat diet, with generous amounts of green, leafy vegetables, whole grains, cottage cheese, yoghurt and buttermilk, cold-pressed oils and a moderate consumption of fruits. Have plenty of pure water, sleep, relaxation and exercise. Encourage breathing to be relaxed and regular.

Deep cleansing is very important. Include steaming and regular mask treatments (as often as three to four times per week) for thorough cleansing and soothing. (Never go outdoors unprotected after using masks.)

Blackheads

These are plugs of sebum and dead cells blocking the mouth of the hair follicle. The sebum oxidizes with the air, turning it black. Often dirt and dust from the air add to the plugs of oil.

TREATMENT – Deep cleansing is essential, but must not damage the acid mantle. Use soaking techniques to slough off dead surface cells. Cleansing grain recipes (page 19) will enable softened blackheads to be removed, without recourse to any harsh peeling or scrubs.

Whiteheads (milea)

These are small, whitish nodules and are the result of trapped oil in the pores, except that a layer of skin covers it. The oil cannot oxidize with the air (turn to blackheads) so it remains white and fatty. Piercing them is likely to scar your skin. Only do so, if you must, after your skin is cleansed and has been softened with steam.

TREATMENT – Keep the skin soft to encourage regeneration. Nourish the area where milea are present. They can be lessened by avoiding sugary, fatty foods which can cause acidic conditions in the body. A balanced diet and regular cleansing will help to gradually reduce their size.

Pimples

Pimples can indicate an increase in hormonal activity or be a symptom of an allergy.

TREATMENT – Do not dry pimples out. Drying the pimple and the surrounding skin tissue can inhibit circulation of nutrients and water, which are needed to activate regeneration processes. Scarring can result. If pimples are inflamed, apply a toner to prevent any more infection and use honey, moor or clay to draw pimple to surface. The same old pimple may recur. To establish the underlying cause, see the Chinese facial chart on page 12.

Broken capillaries

Broken capillaries (veins) show up as fine red lines on cheeks and nose, mostly in a dry, sensitive skin condition or on a thin skin. They can become swollen and congested.

CAUSES – They can be reactions to stimulants such as tea, coffee, alcohol, hot spicy foods, which are able to deplete the body of vitamin C. Even sudden hot and cold changes in your home, such as walking from a warm fire to a cold room, can worsen the condition.

TREATMENT – Protect the area at all times from wind, cold and sun. Always use protection during a steam bath or mask too. It may be best to omit a steam bath altogether, or use for only 3 minutes or less. It is important to keep your system cool and drink plenty of water. Eat sensibly and include vitamin-rich foods. Vitamin C and A can be helpful to strengthen capillary walls (aromatherapeutic essential oils such as cypress, lemon and neroli will also do the same). If there is heat and inflammation, try compressing the skin with lukewarm face towels with added essential oils.

Acid condition

Can appear as patches around the mouth or over the face. Whiteheads can also be present. Skin is sensitive. Acidic disturbances in the skin and body can reactivate such problems as eczema, dermatitis and psoriasis.

CAUSES – Tense muscles of the body can build up stress to cause acidity (see Allergy, page 58). A balance of sodium and potassium (acid/alkaline) in the body is essential, otherwise metabolic disturbance and allergies may result.

TREATMENT – Use rich, medicinal creams or gels to soothe and protect the skin from infection and scarring. Avoid cortisone-based creams. There are natural alternatives available for reducing inflammation without possible long-term side effects.

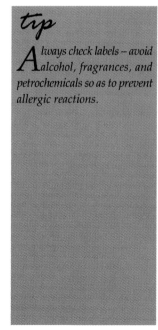

tip

Always check labels – avoid alcohol, fragrances, and petrochemicals so as to prevent allergic reactions.

As with allergic conditions, you should avoid too much protein, alcohol, fried foods, salt and sugar. Eat alkaline-based foods containing potassium (such as green, leafy vegetables, asparagus and bananas) rather than acid ones (such as bread, cheese, raw apples and milk) and avoid excessive tea and coffee. Start each morning by drinking half a lemon squeezed into water.

Allergy

Allergies can appear as mild redness and irritation of the skin and scalp, itching, swelling, coloured boils or pimples. Skin will become sensitive with such reactions and need extra protection. There are two ways that allergies present themselves on the skin.

Firstly, allergies can occur when certain foods or substances are over-consumed over a period of time. This does not allow the delicate cells and enzymes of the body to rest. The organs become sluggish and unable to digest the same foods or substances as well as before. As the system becomes more stressed, over-acidity occurs, producing a reaction as it is eliminated through the skin. The other eliminative organs, such as the liver and kidneys, are also working overtime and may be toxic as well.

Secondly, certain substances are inclined to produce allergic reactions. Pollen and dust in the air are good examples, as are various skincare preparations, petrochemical derivatives, or natural ingredients such as lanolin, cocoa butter, cornstarch, cottonseed oil and many more.

CAUSES – It is most important that the offending substances are identified. Allergies can occur within 10 to 20 minutes of eating food or applying a substance. Sometimes reactions occur straight away, for example from a perfume, making the cause obvious. To test a substance, apply a drop to gauze of bandage and place it on the inner surface of upper arm. (Soap, shampoos and cleansers should first be diluted with water to a concentration as low as 1 part product to 50 parts water.) Check skin under bandage 24 hours later. If it is difficult to detect allergens, consult your practitioner.

TREATMENT – Once an allergen is identified, it is best avoided for about 12 weeks. You may then gradually reintroduce the allergen if you want to. Once your system has had time to regenerate those tired cells and enzymes, be careful not to go back into old habits of eating or applying your potential allergen every day. A balanced diet will provide variety.

To prevent an allergy – become more aware of the difference between needs and habits. Once you start to crave a particular food too often, cut it down from every day to only every three days.

Scarring

CAUSES – Scarring has many causes ranging from birthmarks, vitiligo (pure white areas), acne, rosacea, chloasma, surgery, injuries, burns, animal bites, broken capillaries. Some scars are present from birth or are sustained in early life. Like acne sufferers, people with scarring tend to be self-conscious. Fresh scars from trauma or surgery, when they look their worst, can have damaging psychological effects.

TREATMENT – Scars can eventually fade – sometimes until they are practically unnoticeable – if the skin is encouraged to regenerate by cleansing, toning and extra protection from sun. Use vitamin E, oil or cream, or aloe vera to treat scar tissue.

Treat your skin condition as sensitive and encourage the skin to normalize. When the skin is strengthened and working well, it will look and feel good. Camouflage with foundation can sometimes be used to reduce the severity of scarring. This will take focus away from the area, still giving an artistic and harmonizing natural look.

Glossary

ABSCESS	localized inflammation
ACID	sour fluid, neutralizes alkali
ADIPOSE	fatty tissue in body
ALKALI	bitter fluid, neutralizes acid
ALLERGEN	substance causing allergy
CAPILLARIES	tiny blood vessels
CAROTENE	yellow pigment
CHLOASMA	blotched skin condition
CORTISONE	hormone assisting healing
DIOXANE	organic liquid
DNA	molecule of inheritance (genes)
ESSENTIAL OIL	fragrant plant extract
ETHYLENE OXIDE	toxic substance
FORMALDEHYDE	toxic organic compound
GLYCOL	organic liquid
HAEMOGLOBIN	red pigment in blood
IMMUNE SYSTEM	fights diseases invading body
LYMPH SYSTEM	cleans body of wastes
MELANIN	brown skin pigment
MELANOCYTES	brown pigment granules
MILEA	whiteheads
N-NITROSAMINES	organic nitrogen substances
OZONE LAYER	atmospheric UV shield
PETROCHEMICAL	petroleum by-product
pH	measure of acidity and alkalinity
PHENOL	organic acid (toxic)
POTASSIUM	common mineral in body
ROSACEA	chronic red acne
SILICA	mineral in body, quartz
SODIUM	common mineral in body, salt
SPLEEN	stores blood, fights disease
STEROL	organic substance
TOXINS	wastes produced by cells
UVA, UVB	ultraviolet rays

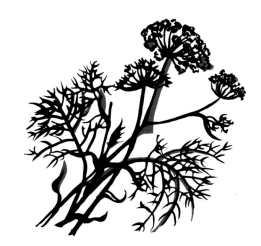

Index